UROGYNAECOLOGY
AND YOU

A Handbook for Women with
Bladder Disorders, Womb and Vaginal Prolapse

UROGYNAECOLOGY AND YOU

A Handbook for Women with Bladder Disorders, Womb and Vaginal Prolapse

Han How Chuan ✎ Lee Lih Charn

Arthur L A Tseng ✎ Wong Heng Fok

KK Women's & Children's Hospital, Singapore

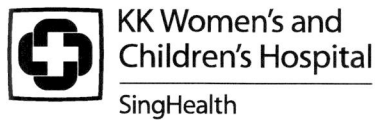

KK Women's and Children's Hospital
SingHealth

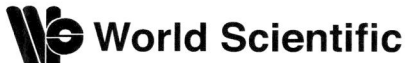

World Scientific

NEW JERSEY · LONDON · SINGAPORE · BEIJING · SHANGHAI · HONG KONG · TAIPEI · CHENNAI

Published by

World Scientific Publishing Co. Pte. Ltd.

5 Toh Tuck Link, Singapore 596224

USA office: 27 Warren Street, Suite 401-402, Hackensack, NJ 07601

UK office: 57 Shelton Street, Covent Garden, London WC2H 9HE

Library of Congress Cataloging-in-Publication Data
Urogynaecology and you : a handbook for women with bladder disorders, womb and vaginal
Prolapse / How Chuan Han .. [et al.].
     p. ; cm.
     Includes index.
     ISBN-13: 978-9814277907 (pbk. : alk. paper)
     ISBN-10: 9814277908 (pbk. : alk. paper)
     1. Genitourinary organs--Diseases--Diagnosis. 2. Urogynecology. I. Han, How Chuan.
     [DNLM: 1. Female Urogenital Diseases--diagnosis. 2. Female Urogenital Diseases--therapy.
     3. Urogenital System. WJ 190 U782 2010]
     RG484.U766 2010
     616.6--dc22

                                                              2009027156

British Library Cataloguing-in-Publication Data
A catalogue record for this book is available from the British Library.

Printed by FuIsland Offset Printing (S) Pte Ltd. Singapore

To our loved ones, friends and colleagues who support and inspire us to greater heights.

Preface

At the beginning of our journey, on 1st April 1990, Kandang Kerbau Hospital (KKH) planted the seed with the start of urogynaecological services. Over the years, this has grown into the present Department of Urogynaecology — a full-fledged and independent department.

Our passion has been to do our very best for our patients, in treating problems like recurrent urinary tract infections, overactive bladder syndrome, stress urinary incontinence, pelvic organ prolapse, painful bladder syndrome, and other urogynaecological problems. To this extent, we have seen our patient numbers increased from a few hundreds in 1990 to more than 12,000 as of 2009.

Advancement in science and medical technology, coupled with improved awareness has resulted in a greater willingness to inquire and explore issues. No longer are patients willing to accept that they must take a prescribed drug to control their problem, or have a particular surgery to cure their medical condition. Modern society has equipped patients with enquiring minds that ask: "Why do I need this medicine, or this particular surgery?" Patients want to be informed on the likelihood of success or improvement for the treatment or surgery they are recommended to take or undergo, and whether there are any complications or side effects. It is with this in mind that we have set out to publish a book that addresses these questions.

We hope that this easy-to-use, concise, yet informative book will help patients understand the common urogynaecological conditions and highlight to them the possible treatment options.

We are truly grateful to all the contributors of this book especially Dr LC Lee and Dr Arthur Tseng who spent much time and effort researching and writing the chapters. We would also like to thank our spouses and families for their support and understanding enabling us to focus in the preparation of this book.

We sincerely thank World Scientific Publishing Co. Ltd. and KK Women's & Children's Hospital for their support during the long process of producing this book and Ms Judy Wong for her dedication and help in liaising between all parties to make this book a reality.

To all our patients who have passed through our doors, and left with a better quality of life and happier hearts, we hereby express our deepest gratitude, appreciation and thanks for your loyal patronage.

We wish you and your family the very best of health always!

Adjunct A/Prof. William Han How Chuan
Head and Senior Consultant
Department of Urogynaecology
KK Women's and Children's Hospital

About the Authors

A/Prof Han How Chuan is a brilliant doctor and surgeon who has pioneered many innovative urogynaecological procedures such as Tension-free Vaginal Tape (TVT), Tension-free Vaginal Tape — Transobturator (TVT-O), and Prolift System in Singapore. He is also a tireless leader who heads the Department of Urogynaecology since 1999. Under his leadership, the Department has flourished in leaps and bounds and the KK Urogynaecology Centre (the first Urogynaecology Centre in the Asia Pacific region) opened its doors on 28 November 2001. A/Prof Han received urogynaecology subspecialty training at St. George's Hospital, United Kingdom in December 1996. He has lectured and published extensively on many urogynaecological conditions. A/Prof Han is a clinical senior lecturer with the NUS Yong Loo Lin School of Medicine and Adjunct Associate Professor of the Duke-NUS Graduate Medical School since August 2008. He is presently Chairman, Section of Urogynaecology, College of Obstetricians & Gynaecologists.

Dr Arthur Tseng is a consultant obstetrician and gynaecologist at KK Women's & Children's Hospital, and has been working there since 1997. Dr Tseng graduated in1996 from Sheffield University and completed his postgraduate studies in 2002. He received further subspecialty training under Professor Linda Cardozo at King's College Hospital, London in 2006. He is actively involved in teaching the Yong Yoo Lin undergraduate medical students and the Duke-NUS postgraduate medical students. Dr Tseng is a frequent contributor of newspaper articles pertaining to women's health issues. He is frequently invited to speak at public forums on urogynaecological issues. Dr Tseng also serves as Honorary Treasurer of The Obstetrical & Gynaecological Society of Singapore and is regarded as an expert in his field by his peers.

Dr Lee Lih Charn is a senior consultant obstetrician and gynaecologist who has worked in KK Women's & Children's Hospital since 1994. She is Head of the Ambulatory and Urodynamics Unit, Department of Urogynaecology. Dr Lee underwent subspecialty training in urogynaecology at St. Vincent's Hospital, Sydney, Australia, in 2000. Her special interests are in patients with urinary incontinence and painful bladder syndrome. Dr Lee has been a clinical senior lecturer with the NUS Yong Loo Lin School of Medicine and Adjunct Assistant Professor of the Duke-NUS Graduate Medical School since August 2008. She has contributed numerous articles to local and international journals on urogynaecology.

Dr Wong Heng Fok is an associate consultant, obstetrician and gynaecologist in KK Women's & Children's Hospital. He has his subspecialty training in urogynaecology at the Royal Women's Hospital, Melbourne, Australia. He has been invited to speak at several public forums and has written articles in international journals on urogynaecology. He is a clinical tutor with the Duke-NUS Graduate Medical School since 2006 and an Adjunct Instructor of the Duke-NUS Graduate Medical School since August 2008.

List of Contributors

Principal Authors

Adj. A/Prof Han How Chuan
Senior Consultant
Obstetrician & Gynaecologist
Head, Urogynaecology Surgery Unit
Head, Department of Urogynaecology
KK Women's & Children's Hospital

Dr Arthur Tseng
Consultant
Obstetrician & Gynaecologist
Department of Urogynaecology
KK Women's & Children's Hospital

Dr Lee Lih Charn
Senior Consultant
Obstetrician & Gynaecologist
Department of Urogynaecology
Head, Ambulatory Care & Urodynamics Unit
KK Women's & Children's Hospital

Dr Wong Heng Fok
Associate Consultant
Obstetrician & Gynaecologist
Department of Urogynaecology
KK Women's & Children's Hospital

Chapter Contributors:

Dr Natalie Chua Weilyn
Medical Officer
Division of Obstetrics & Gynaecology
KK Women's & Children's Hospital

Dr Thanapan Choobun
Clinical Fellow
Department of Urogynaecology
KK Women's & Children's Hospital

Dr Fernandi Moegni
Clinic Fellow
Department of Urogynaecology
KK Women's & Children's Hospital

Dr Arlene Liao
Clnical Fellow
Department of Urogynaecology
KK Women's & Children's Hospital

Contents

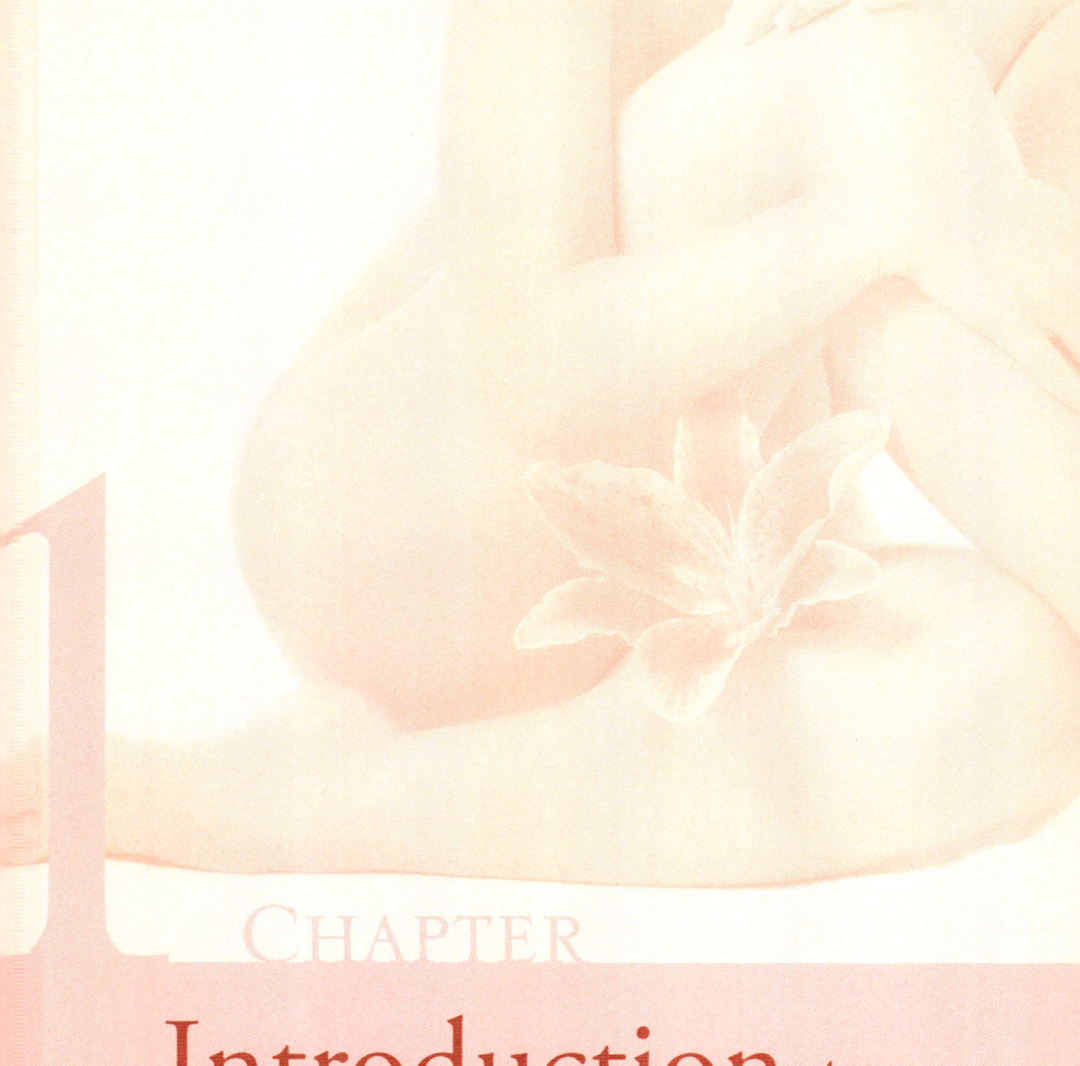

CHAPTER

Introduction to Urogynaecology

What is Urogynaecology (Uro-gy-ne-co-lo-gy)?

The word "**Urogynaecology**" is made up of three parts. The first part "uro" describes the urinary tract, "gynaeco" comes from the Greek word "gyno" which refers to a woman or the female sex, and "logy" comes from the Greek word "logia" which means study.

In brief, urogynaecology is the study of the female urinary and genital tract. It is a sub-specialisation in the field of gynaecology which addresses female bladder problems and pelvic floor dysfunction.

Doctors specialising in this field are known as urogynaecologists. They are obstetricians and gynaecologists who have undergone further training in urogynaecology and pelvic reconstructive surgery.

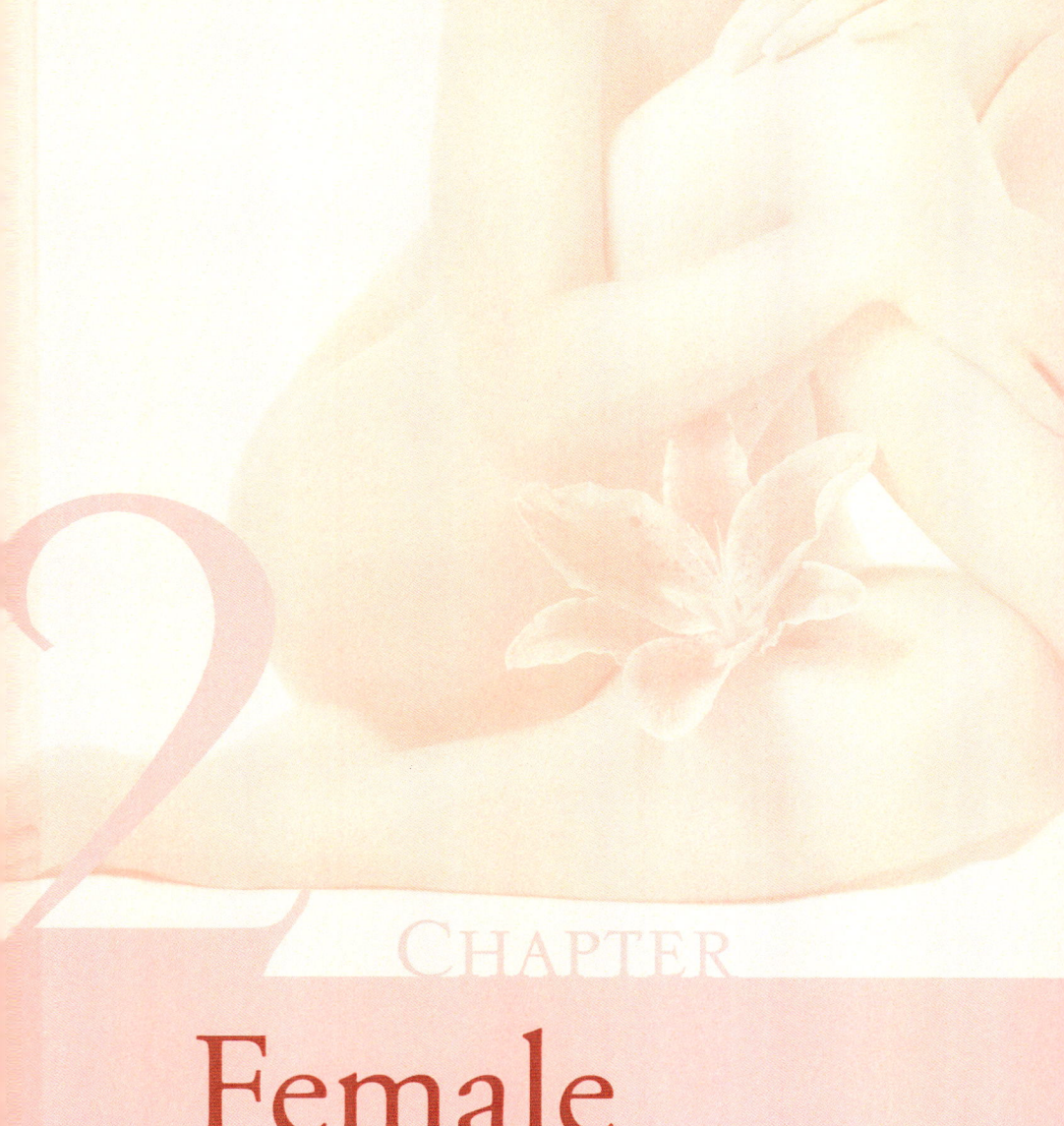

2

Female
Pelvic and Urinary Tract
Anatomy

Female Pelvic Anatomy

The female pelvic organs consist of the vagina, uterus, bladder, urethra, and rectum (Fig. 2.1). All these organs are enclosed in a protective cage called the bony pelvis (Fig. 2.2).

The vagina is the birth canal, which the baby passes through during delivery. It is also the organ used during sexual intercourse, where the male's penis enters the vagina to deposit semen during ejaculation.

The uterus is also called the womb, where a baby develops during pregnancy, and awaits labour to occur.

The bladder is the organ that stores urine, which is continually produced by our kidneys (Fig. 2.3). At suitable occasions where there is privacy, like in the toilet, the bladder expels the stored urine.

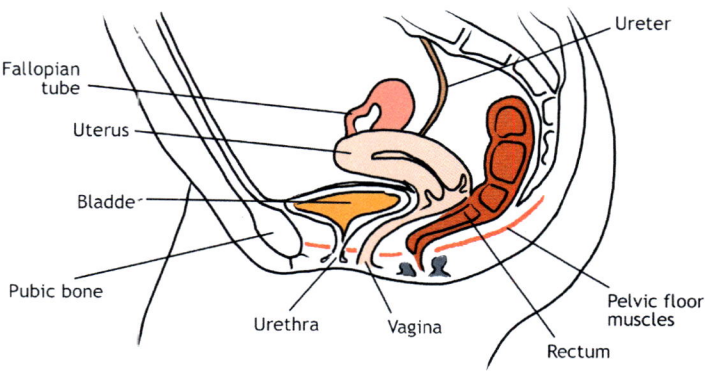

Fig. 2.1.   Side view of the normal female pelvic anatomy.

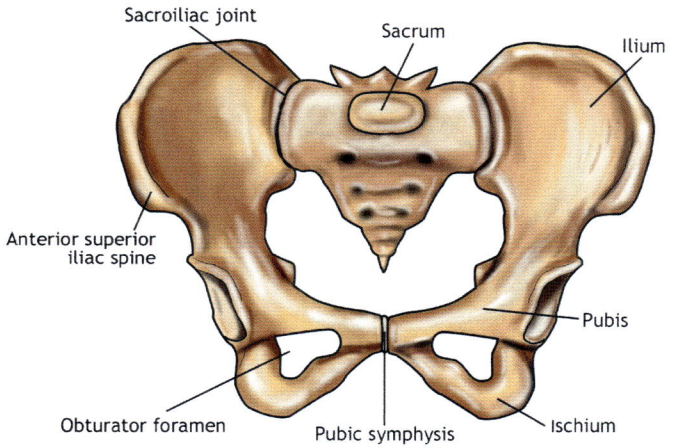

Fig. 2.2. Front view of the normal bony pelvis.

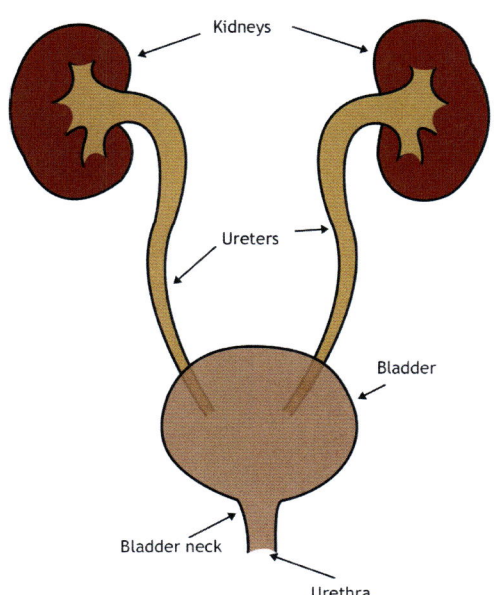

Fig. 2.3. Front view of the urinary tract.

The urethra, otherwise called the "urine tube", is a muscular tube that allows us control over our bladder; such that, at inappropriate times, we can delay passing urine out of the body, and when appropriate, we can "relax" the urethra to empty urine from our bladder.

The rectum is the final portion of the large intestine that stores faecal matter until there is an appropriate situation to expel faeces through the anus.

The condition, when these organs prolapse, is collectively known as pelvic organ prolapse.

3

An Overview of Urogynaecological Conditions

"Doctor, what sort of problem do I have?"

Urogynaecology is a branch of medicine that deals specifically with female bladder disorders and pelvic floor dysfunction. The common symptoms are abnormal frequency of urination, urinary leakage, vaginal and pelvic heaviness or pain, and prolapse of the female pelvic organs.

What are the Common Urogynaecological Conditions?

- Pelvic Organ Prolapse (Chapter 5)
- Stress Urinary Incontinence (Chapter 7)
- Frequency-Urgency Syndrome, or better known as Overactive Bladder (Chapter 8)
- Voiding Disorders, which include slow urination, inability to pass urine, or intermittent flow of urine (Chapter 9)
- Painful Bladder Syndrome (Chapter 10)
- Urinary Tract Infection and Recurrent Urinary Tract Infection (Chapter 11)
- Haematuria (Chapter 12)

This list is not exhaustive. As more women step forward to have their urinary problems investigated and treated, doctors learn more about the disease processes behind each condition.

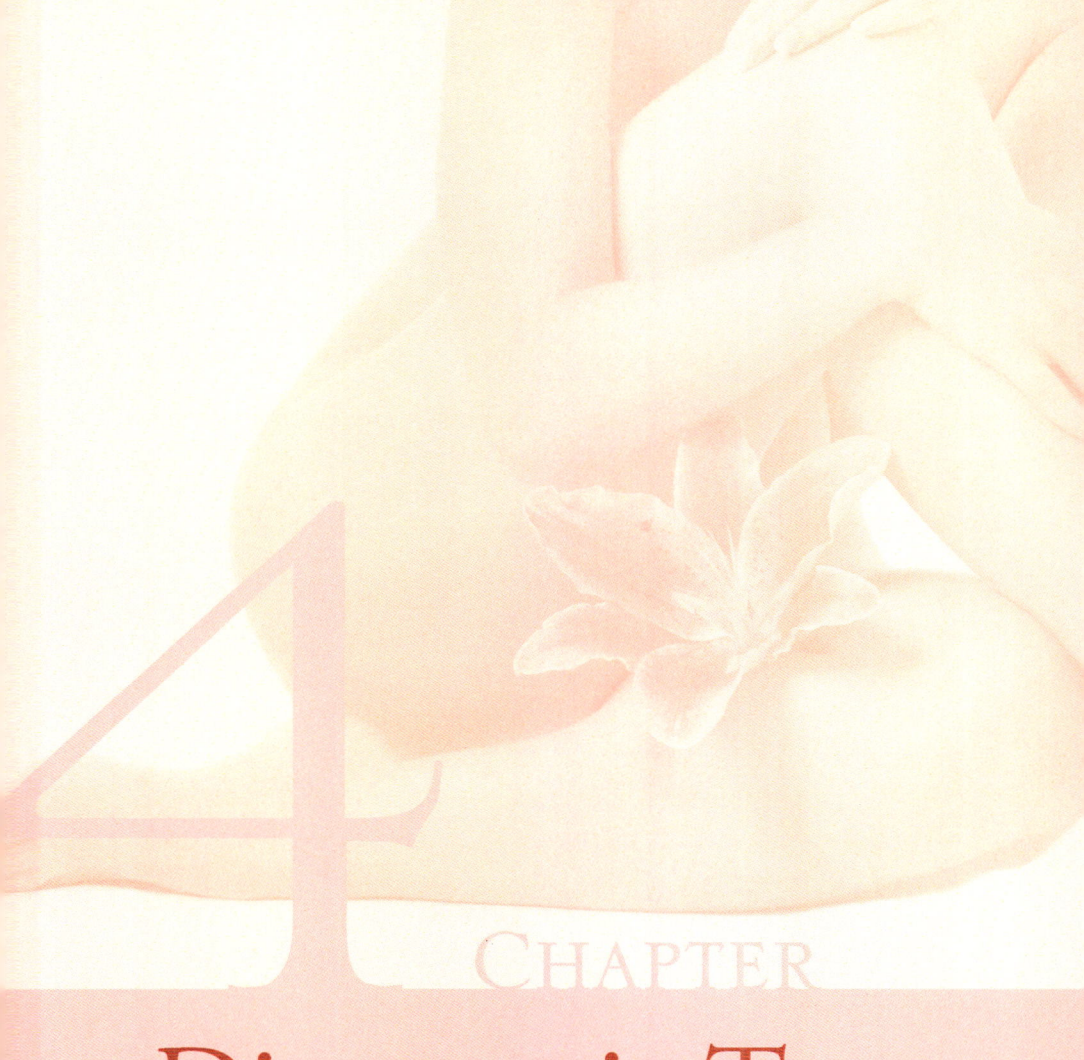

Diagnostic Tests
and Investigations Used
in Urogynaecology and
Urodynamics Studies

"What do I need to undergo to know more about my problem?"

Diagnostic Tests and Investigations

As part of the evaluation of a patient, a detailed history and clinical examination is performed to assess the general medical status of the patient, and decide whether certain medical conditions may affect urinary symptoms. For example, a patient with poorly controlled diabetes mellitus may have troublesome thirst, urinary frequency, disruption of sleep due to frequent urination (nocturia), an overwhelming sensation to pass urine (urgency) and so on.

A detailed urogynaecological examination would involve the assessment of atrophic vaginitis which affects the quality and condition of the vaginal skin. A supine cough test is used to assess stress urinary incontinence, and an erect stress test (EST) can be used as a semi-quantitative test to assess the severity of urinary leakage. An assessment for prolapse of the female pelvic organs is also made. The degree of prolapse of the bladder (cystocoele), rectum (rectocoele), uterus (utero-vaginal prolapse), vaginal vault (vault prolapse), or combinations of pelvic organ prolapse should be made, to decide whether conservative treatment or surgery is needed.

The following tests may be done as part of the initial assessment of the patient:

- Bedside bladder scan
- Dipstick urinalysis
- Urine microscopy and culture
- Ultrasound pelvis
- Ultrasound kidney, ureter and bladder
- Plain abdominal X-ray (AXR)
- Urine cytology
- Cystoscopy with/without biopsy
- Computer tomography (CT) scan
- Intravenous pyelography or urography (IVP/IVU)

A urine dipstick test is a rapid screening test that detects blood (haematuria), sugar (glycosuria) or protein (proteinuria) in the urine and other signs of a urine infection.

A urine microscopy is a test that detects white blood cells, red blood cells, skin cells, nitrites, proteins, micro-organisms, casts and crystals. It is frequently combined with a urine culture for the diagnosis of urinary tract infection (UTI).

A urine culture is used to grow and detect the specific type of bacteria that may be causing a UTI. It also identifies which specific antibiotic can be used to best treat the UTI.

A urine cytology is used to identify suspicious-looking or cancerous cells, which may come from anywhere along the urinary tract. A positive cytology requires urgent assessment with a cystoscopy or other tests, for example, a CT scan.

An ultrasound pelvis is performed to assess the uterus, the fallopian tubes, and the ovaries of the patient. This is to diagnose any masses, such as uterine fibroids or ovarian cysts and tumours, which may cause pressure effects leading to problematic urinary symptoms or prolapse symptoms.

An ultrasound kidney is used to detect renal cysts or masses. A swollen kidney (hydronephrosis) and swollen ureter (hydroureter) can also be visualised with ultrasound. These conditions can be due to internal obstruction, such as stones or tumours in the urinary tract, or external compression, from severe uterine or bladder prolapse.

An abdominal X-ray (AXR) is done to detect stones along the urinary tract. Large staghorn calculi, which look like branches of coral, can occur in the kidneys, whereas smaller stones can occur in the ureters or the bladder.

Cystoscopy involves a specialised endoscopic camera which can be inserted into the bladder to detect chronic infection, bladder stones, foreign bodies, and most importantly, cancerous tumours. Biopsies are samples of tissues taken for definitive diagnosis of chronically inflamed bladder (like painful bladder syndrome) or cancerous tumours (like bladder cancer).

A CT scan is a specialised X-ray test that examines in detail the entire urinary tract after the injection of a dye into a vein. It can diagnose stones, cysts, masses (benign or malignant) and any other abnormalities of the urinary tract; such as extra kidneys, extra ureters, abnormal connections (fistulae) of the urinary tract to other organs, or even an abnormally located kidney (pelvic kidney).

An intravenous pyelogram or urogram (IVP/IVU) is a form of X-ray test, used traditionally to detect any cancerous growths, stones, obstructions in the urinary system, or other abnormalities (like extra kidneys, ureters and so on). With the widespread use of ultrasound and CT scanning today, this test is used less often now.

One particular set of tests, Urodynamic Studies, will be elaborated on below.

Urodynamic Studies

What are urodynamic studies?

These are tests that look at how the bladder and urethra function in relation to each other to store and release urine at appropriate times. It includes uroflowmetry, filling/voiding cystometry and urethral pressure profilometry. These simple tests take about 20 to 30 minutes to complete in a urodynamics facility (Fig. 4.1).

At the start of this series of tests, the patient will be asked to urinate into a commode (uroflowmeter) designed to measure the volume of urine passed, and the speed of urine flow (calculated electronically as millilitres of urine passed per second). Both the average and maximum flow rates are measured. This is uroflowmetry.

Cystometry involves the insertion of fine tubes (catheters) (Fig. 4.2) into the patient's bladder and rectum using an aseptic technique to monitor the pressure changes in her bladder and abdomen while the bladder is being filled with sterile normal saline. After insertion of the catheters, the residual urine is immediately measured to see if the patient's bladder has been completely emptied.

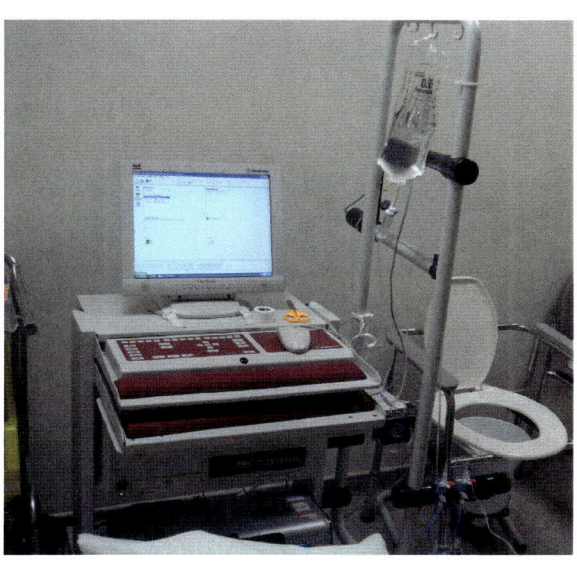

Fig. 4.1. Urodynamic study equipment.

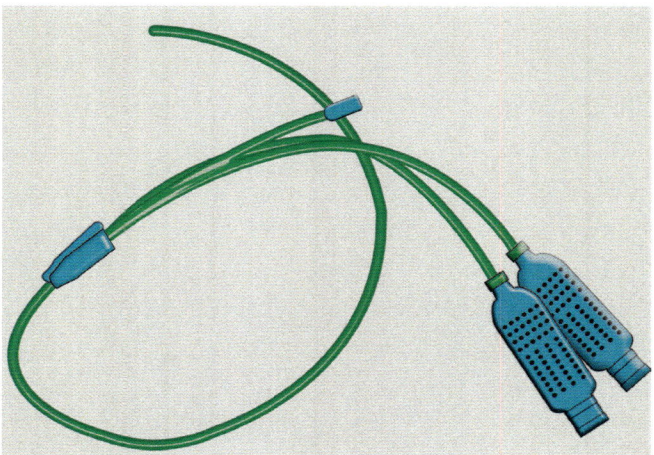

Fig. 4.2. Cystometry catheter.

A trained nurse will attend to the patient throughout the test. The patient will be asked if she has any sensation to pass urine as the bladder is slowly being filled. She will also be required to cough a few times during the procedure. At the end of the test, the patient will be asked to pass urine and empty her bladder over a uroflowmeter again, so that the urine flow in relation to the bladder pressures generated can be assessed.

The time taken for the patient to begin voiding, as well as the force and continuity of the urinary stream will be recorded. The amount of urine passed out, the total time taken to empty the bladder, any straining, hesitancy or dribbling that occurs will also be detected by the machine. Once the test is completed, all catheters will be removed.

The series of test is now complete unless the patient has stress urinary incontinence. If so, an additional test called "Urethral Pressure Profilometry" may be performed to assess the closing pressure of the urethra. This is important because a low closing pressure may decrease the cure rate of continence surgery.

Why does the patient need to take these tests?

These tests are required to understand bladder function and aid in the diagnosis. Especially for patients with complex urinary symptoms, patients due for surgery, or patients who still have problematic urinary symptoms after medical or surgical treatment.

What information will these tests provide?

These tests will provide useful information for the accurate diagnosis and treatment of conditions such as:

- Urodynamic stress incontinence (USI)
- Overactive bladder (OAB)
- Voiding disorders (VD)

What happens after the procedure?

The patient will be given two tablets of antibiotics to be taken immediately after the procedure to lessen UTI occurrence. In addition, she will be advised to drink more water for the day.

The results of the test will be analysed and explained to the patient by the doctor and appropriate treatment can be given.

Are there any complications arising from the procedure?

These are minimally invasive tests and well-tolerated by most patients. UTI is a rare complication, occurring in 3% of patients. This can be minimised by strict adherence to sterile procedural techniques and by taking the preventive antibiotics given immediately after the procedure.

What should the patient look out for after the procedures?

The patient should inform her doctor or go to KK Hospital's 24-hour clinic if she experiences symptoms of UTI. These would include pain when passing urine (dysuria), frequency of urination, nocturia, urgency or supra-pubic pain after the procedure.

Other investigations performed for lower urinary tract dysfunction

Micturating cystourethrogram

Also referred to as a MCU or cystogram, this diagnostic X-ray test helps determine the bladder capacity and the emptying ability of the patient. It also detects abnormalities of the urethra and the bladder. Apart from that, this test can detect a narrowing of the urethra (stricture) secondary to infection or physical trauma, reflux (back-flow) of urine up the ureters during voiding, as well as bladder fistula (an abnormal connection between bladder and another organ).

A MCU is usually performed at the hospital's radiology department. There is no special preparation required of the patient prior to the test. During the procedure, the patient is asked to lie on her back and remain still. A preliminary film of the abdomen area and pelvis is initially done without contrast (dye). This helps the radiologist determine the proper radiographic technique to be used and the positioning of the patient. A catheter is inserted through the urethra into the bladder so that dye can be injected. As the bladder is filled with dye, X-rays of the area in various positions and time intervals are taken. Then, the catheter is removed and additional X-rays are taken as the patient urinates into a container. Once the bladder is emptied, a final X-ray is taken. The entire test takes approximately an hour to complete.

5

CHAPTER

Pelvic Organ Prolapse

"Doctor, something is sticking out of my vagina!"

Introduction

With recent major advances in medical care, many chronic diseases can now be managed successfully, and women's healthcare has greatly improved. However, in our longer-living but rapidly ageing population, the problems associated with ageing are also becoming more common.

One common problem that affects a woman's quality of life is pelvic organ prolapse (POP). POP is common, nearly 45% of menopausal women suffer from some degree of the condition. Fortunately, POP can be treated with a variety of methods.

The pelvic organs consist of the uterus (womb), bladder, urethra, rectum (gut), and vagina (Fig. 5.1) of which any can prolapse.

What is Pelvic Organ Prolapse?

A prolapse is the protrusion of an organ beyond its normal position. The protrusion of the uterus (womb) along the axis of the vagina, or out of it is called utero-vaginal prolapse (UVP) (Fig. 5.2). The commonest form of prolapse in women is a prolapse of the bladder and the urethra, which presents as a protrusion of the anterior vaginal wall (cystourethrocoele) (Fig. 5.3). Other types of prolapse include a protrusion of the rectum from the posterior vaginal wall (rectocoele) (Fig. 5.4).

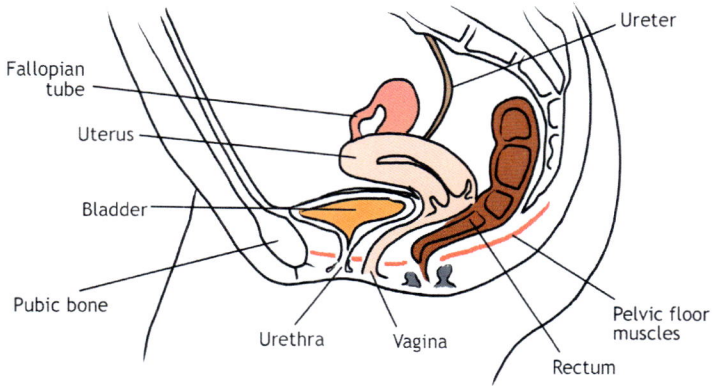

Fig. 5.1. Side view of normal female pelvic anatomy.

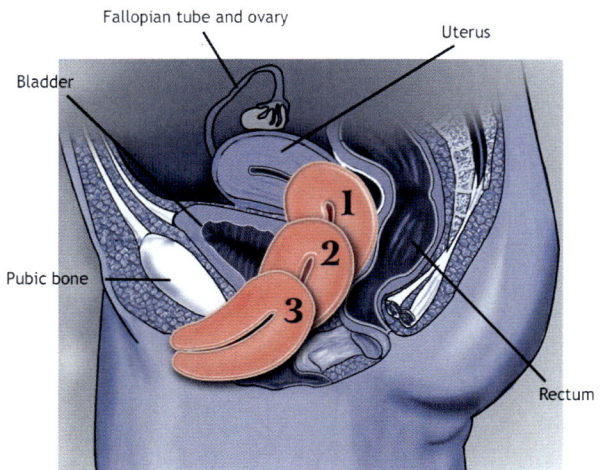

Fig. 5.2. The three degrees of utero-vaginal prolapse —
describing severity of prolapse.

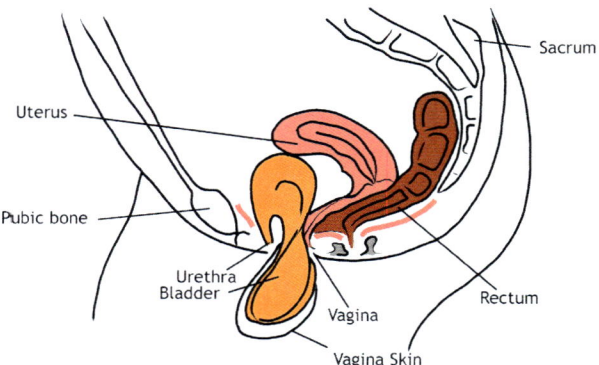

Fig. 5.3. Cystourethrocoele — a protrusion of the bladder with the anterior vaginal wall.

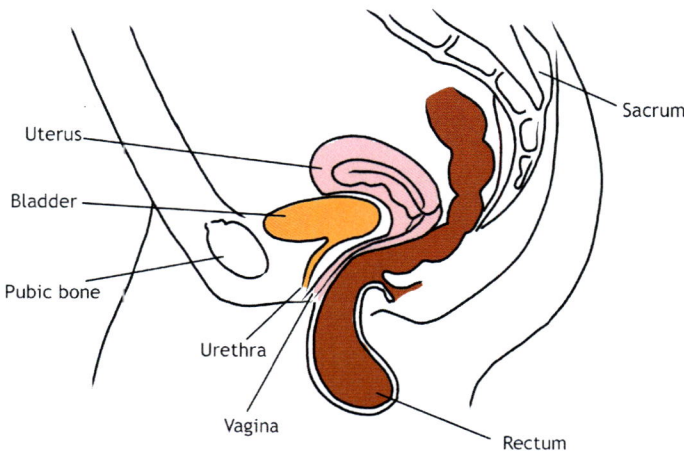

Fig. 5.4. Rectocoele — a protrusion of the rectum from the posterior vaginal wall.

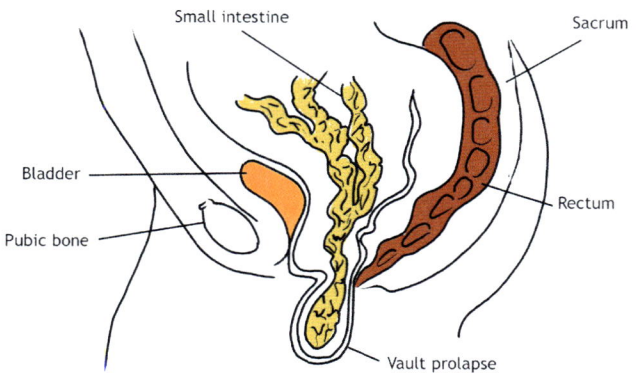

Fig. 5.5. Vault prolapse — the vagina everts outwards through the vaginal introitus.

In cases where the womb has been removed, the rest of the vagina can still prolapse (vault prolapse) (Fig. 5.5).

What are the Various Types of Pelvic Organ Prolapse?

• Cystocoele (bladder prolapse)

When the bladder prolapses, it pushes itself through the vagina and creates a large bulge through the front vaginal wall. It is common for both the bladder and the urethra to prolapse together. This is called a cystourethrocoele and is the most common type of prolapse in women (Fig. 5.6).

• Rectocoele (rectal wall prolapse)

This occurs when the end of the large bowel (rectum) loses support and bulges through the back wall of the vagina (Fig. 5.7). It is different from a rectal prolapse (when the rectum protrudes through the anus).

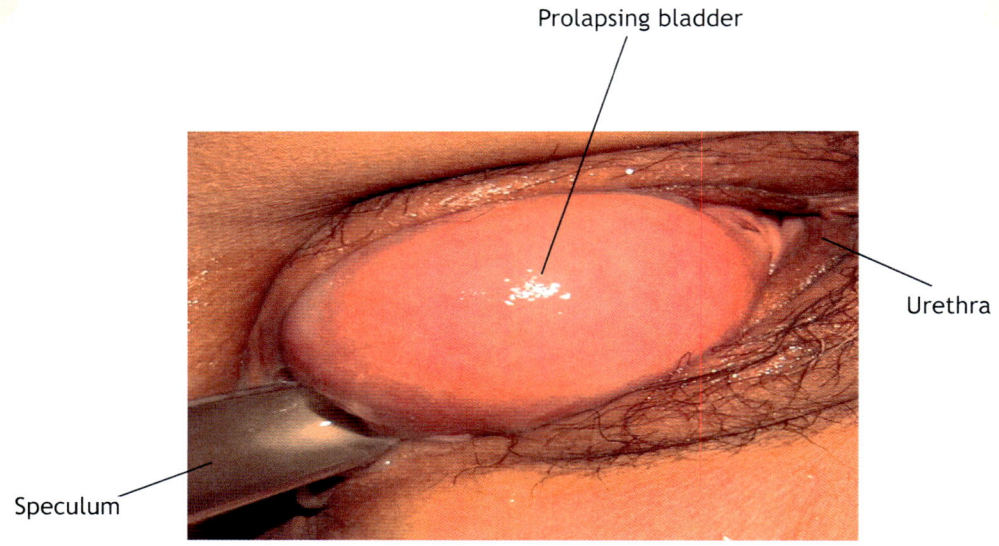

Fig. 5.6.   Cystourethrocoele — patient lying down on her left-side while straining down.

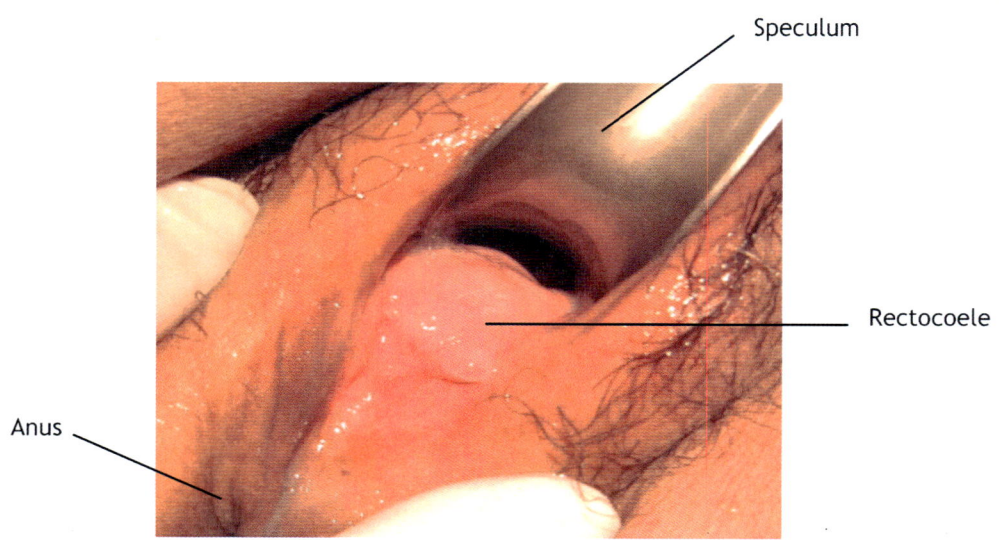

Fig. 5.7.   Rectocoele — patient lying down on her left-side while straining down.

- ### Enterocoele (prolapse of the small bowel)

In this case, part of the small intestine in the pouch of Douglas may slip down between the rectum and the back wall of the vagina (Fig. 5.8). This often occurs at the same time as a rectocoele or uterine prolapse.

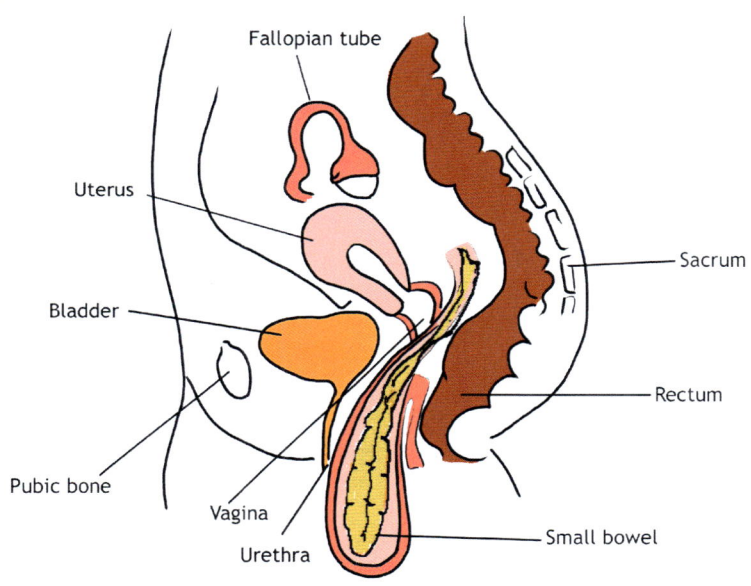

Fig. 5.8. Enterocoele — Small bowel prolapse.

- ### Uterine prolapse

Uterine prolapse is when the womb drops down the vagina (Fig. 5.9). It is the second most common type of prolapse. The severity of the prolapse is described in three degrees: a first-degree uterine prolapse being very mild and asymptomatic and, a third-degree uterine prolapse being the most severe (Fig. 5.10). It is also called a procidentia.

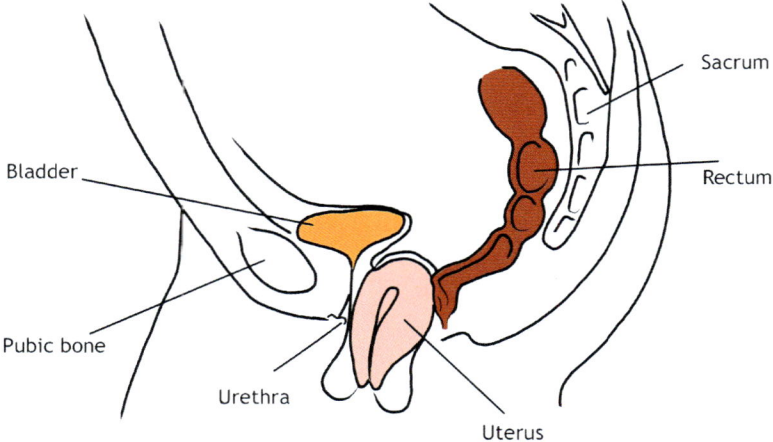

Fig. 5.9.   Severe uterine prolapse with chronic swelling of overlying vaginal skin.

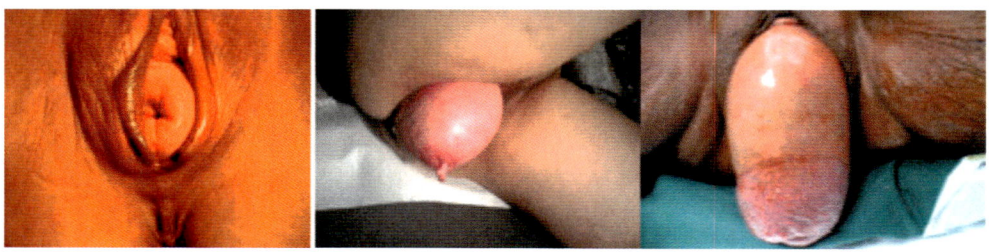

Fig. 5.10.   Examples of severe uterine prolapse — 2nd degree, 3rd degree and a procidentia (from left to right).

- ## Vaginal vault prolapse

The vaginal vault is the apex of the vagina. It can fall in on itself after a woman's uterus has been removed (hysterectomy). Vault prolapse occurs in about 5% of women who have had a hysterectomy (Fig. 5.5).

Grades of Pelvic Organ Prolapse

Four grade levels are used to describe the severity of POP.

Grade 0: There is no prolapse of any of the pelvic organs, and it is usually found in women who have never delivered children before (Fig. 5.11).

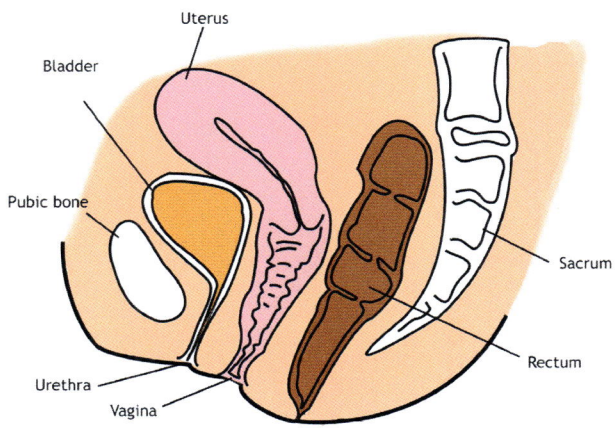

Fig. 5.11.   No prolapse.

Grade 1: The organ has dropped slightly. At this stage, the prolapse is asymptomatic, and is an incidental finding during a gynaecological examination (Fig. 5.12).

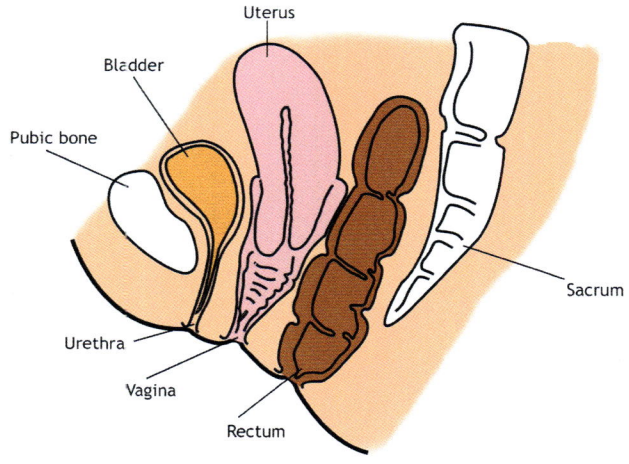

Fig. 5.12.   Grade 1 prolapse of the uterus.

Grade 2: The organ has dropped further into the vagina towards the introitus. It can be associated with symptoms of heaviness, and possibly the feeling of something in the vagina during cleansing of the region (Fig. 5.13).

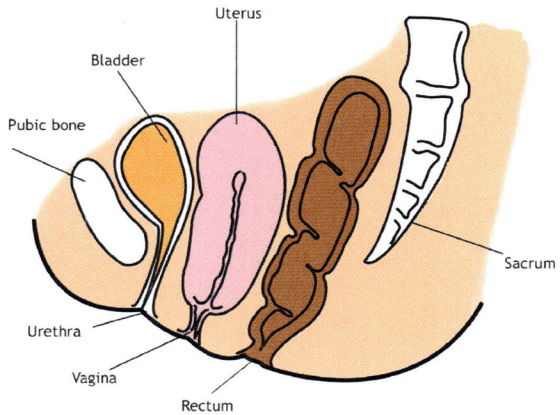

Fig. 5.13.   Grade 2 prolapse of the uterus.

Grade 3: A significant portion of the organ has fallen through the vaginal opening, and can be seen protruding from the vaginal opening (Fig. 5.14).

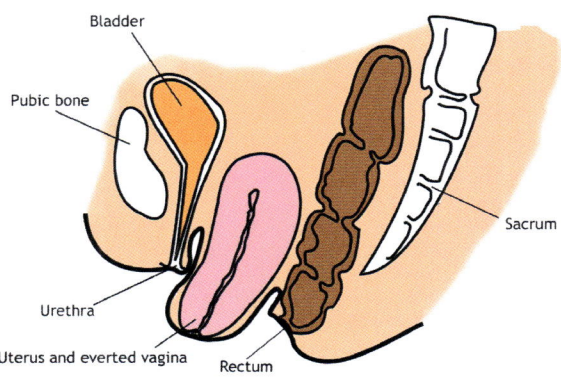

Fig. 5.14.   Grade 3 prolapse of the uterus.

Grade 4: The whole organ has completely fallen through the vaginal opening. This is the most severe form of prolapse. It is specifically called a procidentia, when the uterus is completely out of the vagina (Fig. 5.15).

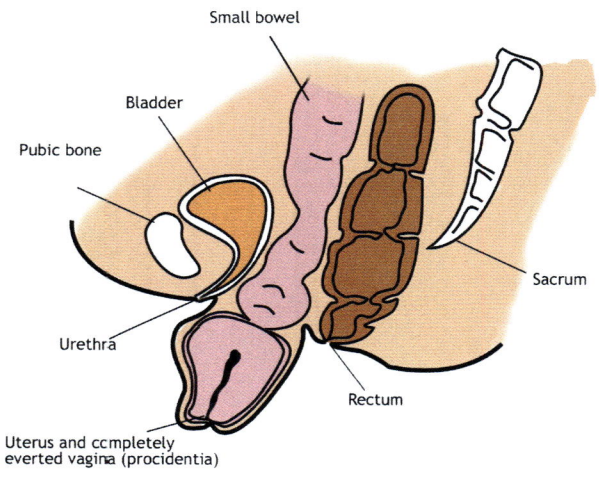

Fig. 5.15.   Grade 4 prolapse of the uterus.

What Causes a Prolapse?

It results from deterioration or relaxation of the supporting tissues (the pelvic floor) around the pelvic organs. There are many risk factors that lead to this pelvic floor relaxation such as pregnancy, vaginal delivery, menopause, and so on.

Some people believe that caesarean sections can prevent POP, but this is only partly true if the woman has one or two caesarean sections. The risk for POP would be the same as in the case of multiple vaginal deliveries if the woman has three or more caesarean sections.

Conditions that increase the pressure in the abdominal cavity can also directly affect the pelvic floor. Prolonged effects of pressure eventually result in a downward displacement of the pelvic organs from their normal position. Chronic cough, asthma, constipation, carrying heavy objects or loads, and obesity are some causative examples of this prolonged pressure effect. Patients who have had previous pelvic surgery are also susceptible to an increased risk of prolapse.

The symptoms and severity of the prolapse usually depends on the degree of prolapse. Symptoms include feeling a sense of heaviness in the vagina, pelvic discomfort, feeling or seeing a protrusion at the vaginal opening, difficulty having sexual intercourse, or feeling low back pain. In severe cases, women may have difficulty passing urine or motion. Some sufferers experience chronic vaginal discharge or bleeding resulting from repeated injury to the prolapsed organ. The patient's symptoms usually improve when she lies down but worsen when she stands for prolonged periods of time.

Patients with severe utero-vaginal prolapse or cystocoele for a long time may have enlarged ureters and kidneys, due to obstruction of the ureter/urethra when it is completely kinked.

Scenario 1

A 60-year-old woman went to see the doctor because she experienced the feeling of vaginal heaviness for a year. One week before her consultation, she felt and discovered a lump in her vagina. She had previously delivered five children, all through natural childbirth and was being treated for asthma and chronic constipation for many years. The doctor performed a speculum examination of her vagina and a pelvic examination. She was diagnosed with a prolapse of the bladder and the womb.

How can a Prolapse be Treated?

Not every patient with POP needs to undergo surgery. The decision to undergo treatment depends on the age, prolapse severity, underlying medical diseases, and whether childbearing has ceased.

There are two treatment options available for POP: conservative and surgical treatments.

Conservative treatment

Generally, when women suffer from prolapse, it is impossible for them to recover on their own. The most popular non-surgical treatment is pelvic floor exercise (PFE) or Kegel exercises. This exercise strengthens the pelvic floor muscles and slows down the progression of the prolapse. The success of PFE depends on how regularly the exercise is carried out. PFE may improve the condition in the short-run but does not cure it, as the prolapse will worsen once PFE is stopped. It is only suitable for milder degrees of prolapse.

Patients with severe POP but who are not suitable for surgery or do not want surgery may have a vaginal pessary fitted. This is done to support the prolapsed organ and relieve their symptoms. Patients who use pessaries (Figs. 5.16(a) and (b)) will require a regular pelvic examination every 3 to

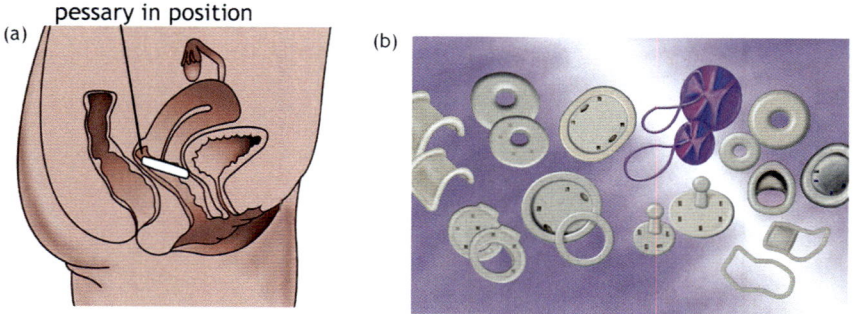

Fig. 5.16.   (a) Pessary placement; (b) various types of vaginal pessaries.

4 months. During examination, the pessary is removed, and the vagina cleansed and checked for any skin erosions or ulcers due to pressure effects. If no skin lesions are noted, the pessary is changed, and a review date is arranged in 3 to 4 months' time.

Surgical treatment

The definitive form of management of POP is surgery. There are many types of operation depending on the patient's condition, the type and severity of POP, and the preference of the patient. A urogynaecologist is best able to discuss with the patient the type of surgery, the risks and complications involved, the anaesthesia required, and the post-operative management.

In the case of a utero-vaginal prolapse, the appropriate treatment would be the removal of womb via the vaginal route (vaginal hysterectomy). If the patient prefers to keep her womb, the surgeon will repair the womb to its normal position. In patients with an elongated cervix, the cervix may need to be removed (Manchester operation).

Women who have vaginal wall prolapse such as a cystourethrocoele or rectocoele can be treated with a pelvic floor repair. This procedure reduces unsightly bulges and discomfort once the normal anatomy has been restored.

For severe POP cases, there is a high chance of recurrent prolapses in the future, especially those who suffer from cystourethrocoele. To decrease the risk of recurrence, the doctor may discuss with the patient about using a synthetic mesh (e.g. Gynemesh Prolift®) (Fig. 5.17) to support the prolapsing organ(s). The mesh is made of non-absorbable material woven into a net, which is placed beneath the vaginal skin and left inside the body for life. The risk of mesh erosion, protruding through the vaginal skin is up to 10%.

For those with vault or severe uterine prolapse, treatment is by a procedure known as sacrospinous ligament fixation, which attaches the vaginal vault to a strong ligament within the pelvis. The most common side effect of this treatment is short-term discomfort/pain in the right buttock region, which can be relieved with painkillers.

Whilst abdominal or laparoscopic surgery is possible, vaginal prolapse surgery has the advantage of absence of a scar on the abdomen and lower level of pain experienced by patients during the post-operative period.

POP is not a life-threatening condition, unlike cancer. It does however, cause patients a great deal of bother, and adversely affects their quality of life. Patients should discuss with their specialists the problems associated with their particular conditions, the treatment options, cure and complication rates of different methods of treatment.

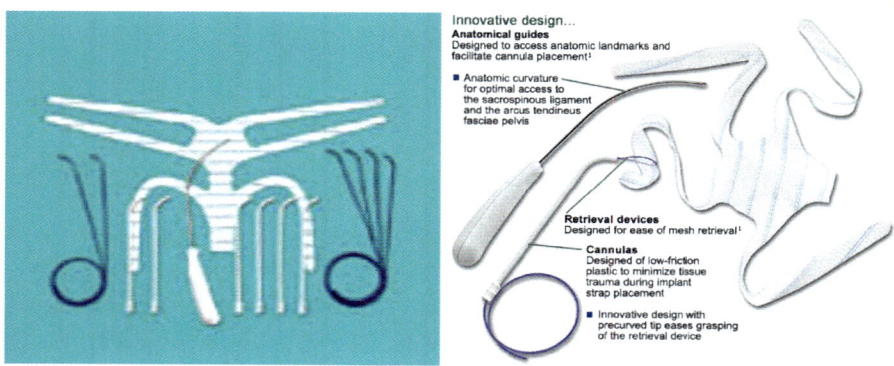

Fig. 5.17.   Prolift" Kit (courtesy of Johnson & Johnson Medical Limited).

Scenario 2

A 60-year-old woman, was diagnosed with a grade 4 utero-vaginal prolapse, a grade 4 cystocoele and a grade 2 rectocoele. Her doctor discussed with her the various treatment options, which included the insertion of a vaginal pessary or surgery. She decided to remove her womb and repair her pelvic floor and vagina. The doctor explained to her about the sacrospinous ligament fixation procedure and the use of a mesh to prevent a recurrent prolapse. She decided to go ahead with the procedure to use the mesh and accepted the small risk of mesh erosion. Before the operation, she was sent for pre-operative blood tests, a chest X-ray and an electrocardiogram (ECG).

Pain Management During and After Operation

The patient is pain-free during surgery due to administration of anaesthesia. This can be broadly divided into two types: general and regional anaesthesia.

The use of general anaesthesia involves the patient being unconscious (sleeping) while the operation is performed. Regional anaesthesia is the method of injecting anaesthetic agents into the spinal space, affecting the nerves, such that the patient loses sensation in her lower body (Fig. 5.18). This method can be used to provide pain relief for as long as is required. The patient is conscious while the doctor performs the surgery. The anaesthetist will discuss with the patient the pros and cons of each type of anaesthesia before the operation.

The traditional postoperative pain relief methods include the use of painkiller injections or oral medications. Other newer methods of pain control include the use of patient controlled analgesia (PCA) pumps, which allow the patient to control the dosage of pain relief medication on her own by pressing a device whenever she requires pain relief.

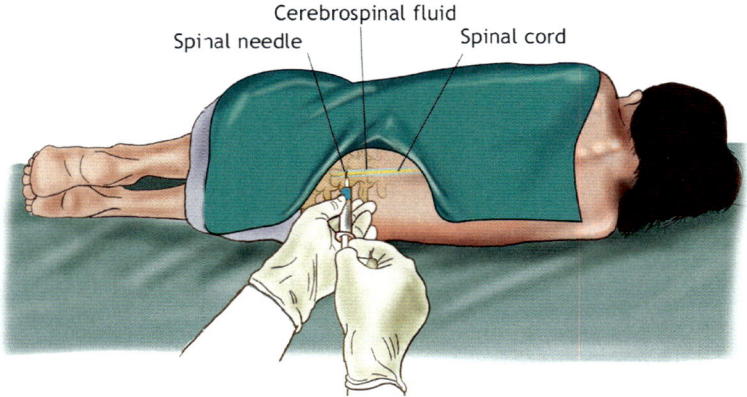

Cerebrospinal fluid

Spinal needle

Spinal cord

Fig. 5.18.   Regional anaesthesia — applying a spinal block.

What are the Complications for Vaginal Surgery?

The complications fall into two categories: anaesthesia-related and surgery-related.

Surgical complications include the risk of bleeding, infection of wound site and trauma to adjacent organs such as the bladder or rectum. In experienced hands, these risks are low (less than 1%). The risk of infection can be drastically reduced by using appropriate antibiotics during surgery.

Some complications do not occur at the wound site, but at other sites. Chest infection can occur in the first few post-operative days. Deep breathing exercises to expand the lungs and early mobilisation can decrease the risk. Urinary tract infection (UTI) can occur post-operatively. Early mobilisation and removal of indwelling catheter reduce the occurrence of UTI.

There is also the risk of blood clots developing in the patient's legs when pelvic surgery is performed. Once the clot develops, it can become life-threatening if the clot dislodges and settles in the lungs, causing obstruction to blood flow and reduced oxygen exchange. The use of graduated pressure stockings called thrombo-embolic deterrent (TED) stockings (Fig. 5.19) and pneumatic calf compressors (Fig. 5.20) can reduce the chance of such complications from developing. In addition, patients are given low molecular heparin injections to deter blood clot formation during the immediate post-operative period.

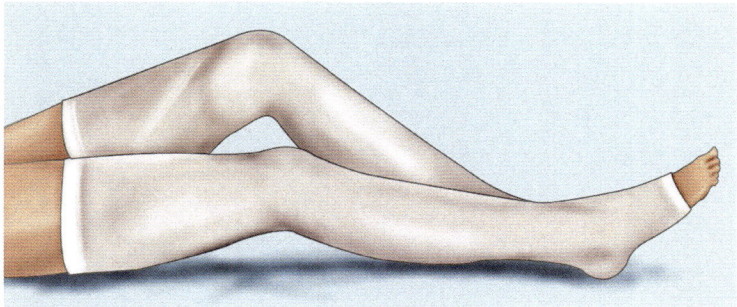

Fig. 5.19. TED stockings.

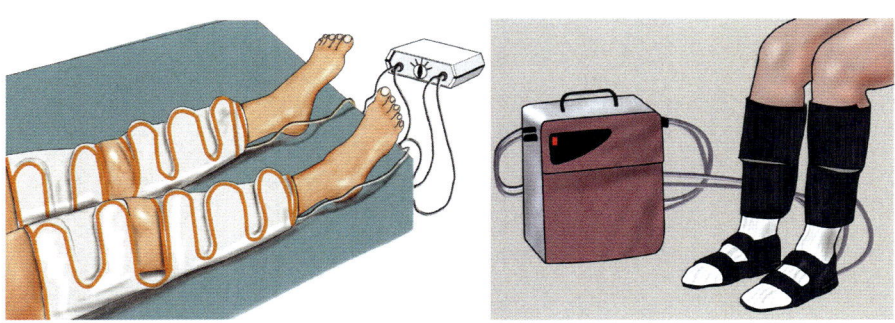

Fig 5.20. Pneumatic cuff compressors.

Scenario 3

A 60-year-old woman, was diagnosed with a grade 3 utero-vaginal prolapse and cystocoele. She had undergone a vaginal hysterectomy, and an anterior Prolift cystocoele repair, under spinal anaesthesia. The operation went smoothly, without complications; and an indwelling catheter and an antiseptic vaginal pack was inserted.

In the ward, the patient was advised to wear the TED stockings all the time, and the pneumatic leg compressor cuffs would be removed the next post-operative day (the TED stockings should be worn for a further 1 week after discharge). She was allowed to eat after the review on the first post-operative day. The bladder catheter and vaginal pack were taken out on the second post-operative day. There was some discomfort during the removal of the pack, but it soon subsided. The doctor reviewed the patient and confirmed that she had not developed any complications, and she went home after being able to pass urine with ease. The patient was given 4 weeks of hospitalisation leave.

Post-operative Care and Follow-up

The patient will be given a review date at the outpatient clinic within one week after surgery. She will be asked if she experiences any symptoms of pain, bleeding from the vagina, fever, as well as how well she is able to pass urine and clear her bowels. If there are no complications, the patient will be advised to return for appointments at intervals of 1 month, 6 months and a year thereafter.

There is always a chance of prolapse recurring after prolapse surgery. Post-operatively, the patient is advised to avoid carrying heavy objects (more than 5 kg) or strenuous activities. The treatment of chronic cough and asthma, and avoidance of constipation are also important. A weight loss programme for obese patients will reduce the chance of a recurrent prolapse. Pelvic floor exercise (PFE) can also help to strengthen the pelvic floor and deter recurrence.

Conclusion

POP is a common problem experienced by women from all walks of life. It is not a life-threatening condition but can adversely affect the quality of life of the sufferer. By reducing risk factors or avoiding certain lifestyle habits, POP can be prevented. One method of prevention is by carrying out pelvic floor exercise, an activity that is not only useful at every stage of a woman's life but also has an added benefit of improving the quality of one's sexual function. If a women has or suspects that she has POP, she should not be embarrassed about consulting her doctor. This condition can be successfully treated with a low complication rate. Early detection and treatment invariably leads to a good outcome.

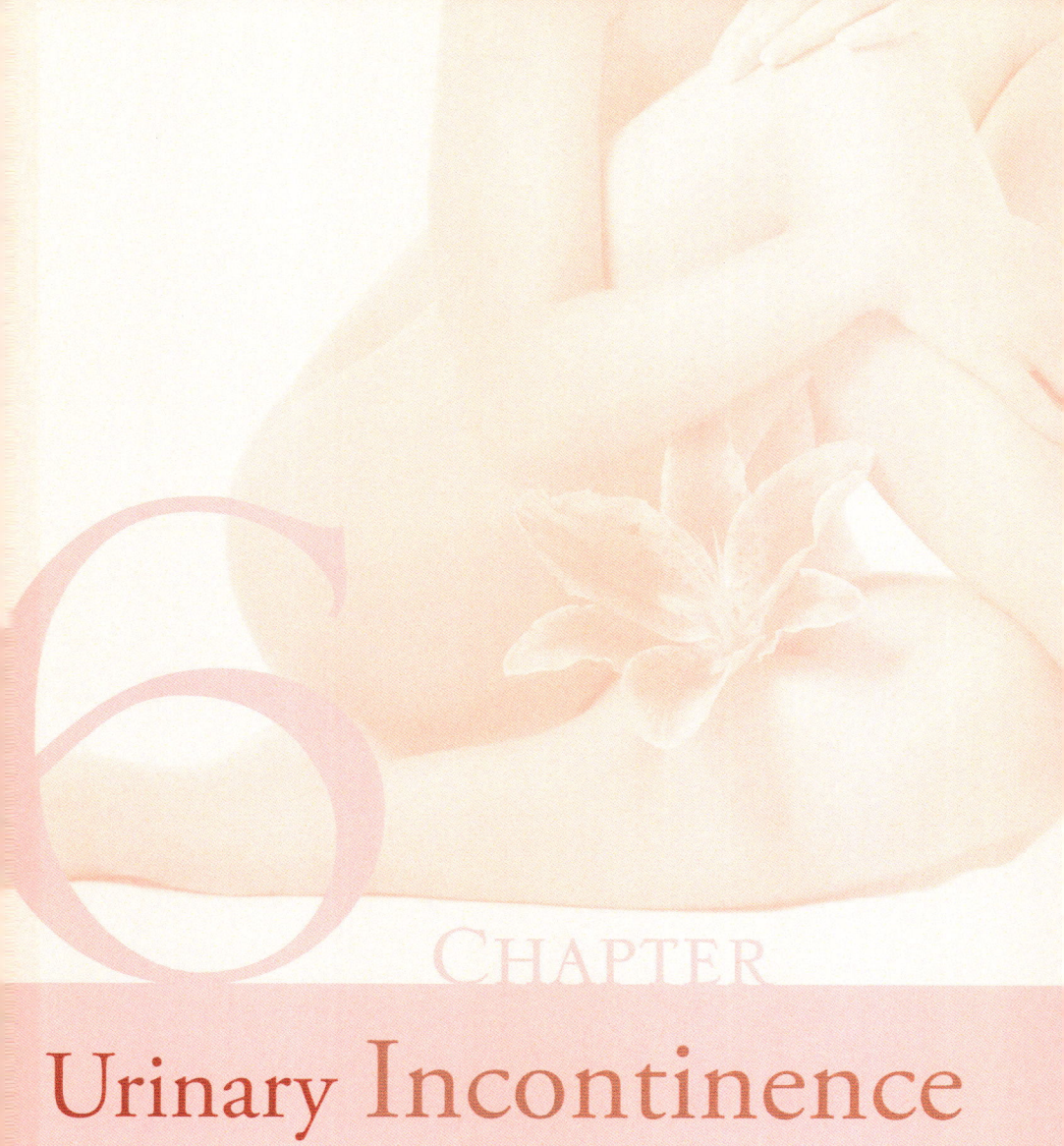

6

CHAPTER

Urinary Incontinence

What is Urinary Incontinence?

Urinary incontinence is the inability to prevent the loss of urine from the bladder. The severity of urinary incontinence can range from an occasional leakage of urine when one coughs or sneezes, to sudden and unpredictable episodes of urine leakage. Sometimes, the incontinence may result from an urgency to urinate and one may not be able to make it to the toilet in time. This is a common troublesome and embarrassing problem that women face (Fig. 6.1).

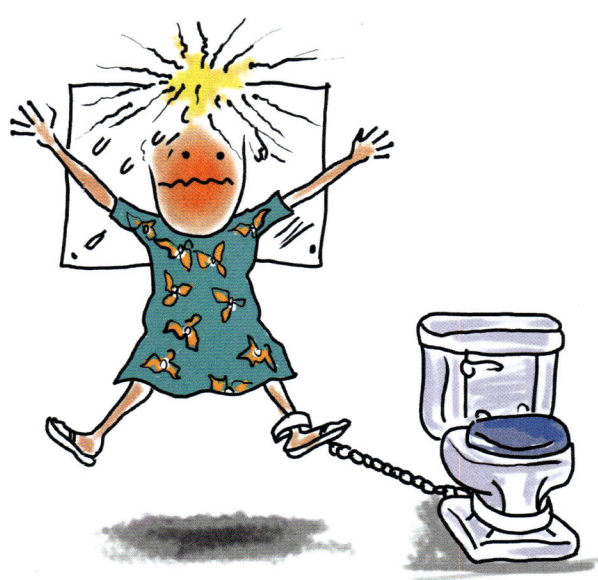

Fig. 6.1.   Urinary incontinence — the distress of being "chained" to the toilet.

"Transient incontinence" is a temporary episode of urinary incontinence. The condition can be triggered by medications, UTI, mental impairment, restricted mobility or severe constipation with stool impaction which obstructs urine flow and subsequently causes an overflow of urine. Incontinence can also simply occur when one works at a task for a long time and postpones going to the toilet for too long.

What are the Types of Urinary Incontinence?

Stress urinary incontinence (SUI)

It is the involuntary leakage of urine triggered by coughing, laughing, sneezing, exercising or other physical exertions that increase the intra-abdominal pressure on the bladder. The problem is more noticeable when the bladder is full. SUI is the most common type of urinary incontinence, affecting 50% of women with urinary leakage. This topic is further discussed in Chapter 7.

Urge incontinence

This involves a sudden, intense need to urinate (urgency). Such a need is difficult to defer, and the urge may be followed by an involuntary loss of urine. To learn more on urge incontinence, please read Chapter 8 on "Frequency-Urgency Syndrome" (Fig. 6.2).

Overflow incontinence

If a patient dribbles urine frequently, she may have overflow incontinence. Overflow incontinence is the inability to empty the bladder due to a weakened or damaged bladder that is overfilled with urine. With overflow incontinence, the patient may have a sensation that she has not completely emptied her bladder after urination. In addition, when she tries to urinate, she may produce only a weak stream of urine.

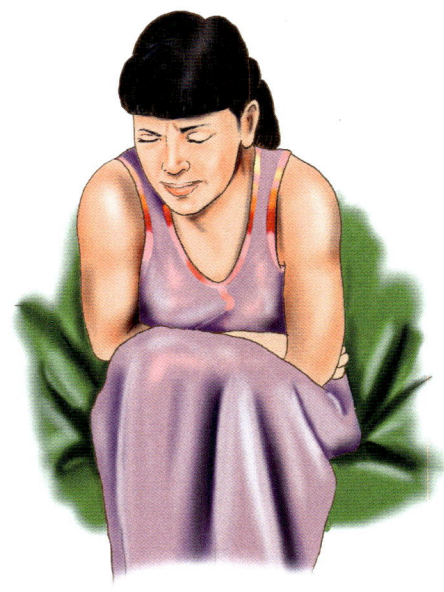

Fig. 6.2. The distress and sense of isolation caused by urgency, frequency of urination and urinary incontinence.

Mixed incontinence

If the patient experiences a combination of stress incontinence and urge incontinence symptoms, she has mixed incontinence. Most of the time, one particular type of urinary incontinence predominates.

True incontinence

True incontinence is caused by a fistula. An urinary fistula is an abnormal connection between the urinary tract and another organ. Fistulae can be due to difficult childbirth, surgery, radiation therapy or certain diseases. An obstetric fistula is usually caused by obstructed labour, when the prolonged pressure of the baby's head against the mother's pelvis cuts off blood supply to delicate tissues in the region.

The tissue dies and breaks down, and a hole forms between the vagina and the bladder (vesicovaginal fistula), or between the vagina and the rectum (rectovaginal fistula) or both. The result is uncontrollable leaking of urine or faeces or both.

Pelvic surgery or radiation therapy are also known to cause vesicovaginal fistulae, while inflammatory bowel diseases, such as Crohn's disease and ulcerative colitis, can cause a fistula between the bowel and vagina.

Occasionally, a patient could be born with a fistula, i.e. a congenital fistula.

Diagnosis of Urinary Incontinence

A careful history-taking is essential to discern the type of urinary incontinence a patient suffers from. Of importance will be issues such as straining and discomfort during urination, the use of medication, previous pelvic surgery and other medical conditions like diabetes mellitus.

The physical examination focuses on ascertaining the symptoms of incontinence. The patient will undergo a general medical examination; a gynaecological and urogynaecological examination, which includes an erect stress test (EST). A nervous system examination may be done in some patients. Other investigations like a bedside ultrasound scan, to estimate bladder residual urine volumes may be done.

A urodynamic study is often performed as a means of differentiating the different types of urinary incontinence. The test will also ascertain the patient's functional bladder capacity and post-void residual urine volume to check for evidence of poorly functioning bladder muscles.

Other tests include:

- Urine microscopy and culture
- Ultrasound of the kidneys, ureters and bladder
- Cystoscopy with or without biopsy

Conclusion

If a patient has trouble controlling her bladder, she should consult her doctor. Urinary incontinence can be cured or at the very least controlled, thus improving quality of life for the patient.

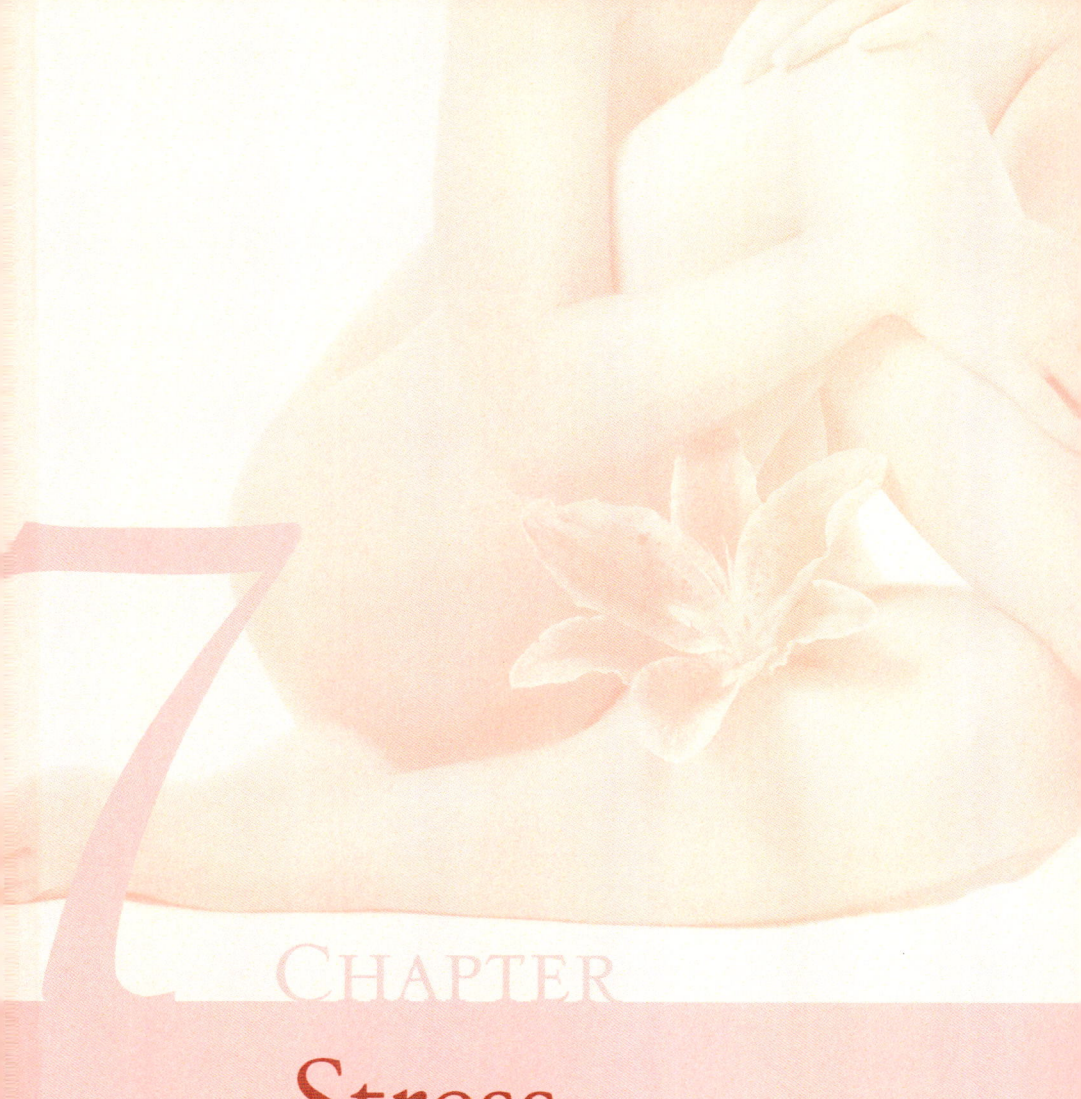

CHAPTER

Stress
Urinary Incontinence

Introduction

If coughing, sneezing, laughing or other physical activities that put pressure on the bladder such as jogging causes a woman to leak urine, she has stress urinary incontinence (SUI).

Urinary incontinence affects about 10 to 20 million American women. Based on a Gallup survey conducted in 2002, up to 70% of the women with incontinence display symptoms attributable to SUI. In the United States alone, SUI affects one in three women over the age of 18 years.

In Singapore, about 15% of women suffer from SUI. Yet many women are too embarrassed to talk about it or discuss it with their doctors due to the stigma associated with SUI, as well as fear of surgery (Fig. 7.1). Instead, most women alter their lifestyles drastically so as to avoid embarrassment, mistakenly assuming that incontinence is a normal part of ageing.

How would a woman know if she suffers from SUI? How could she deal with it? She could consult her doctor, a gynaecologist or a urogynaecologist to find out more.

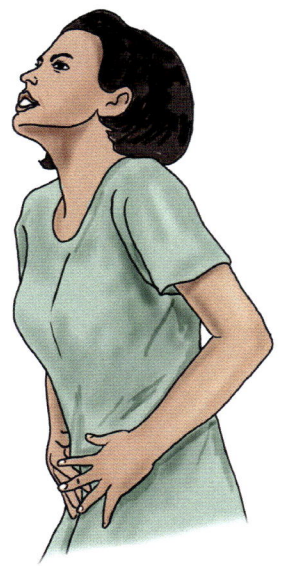

Fig. 7.1. Stress urinary incontinence — an embarrassing and distressing condition for women.

What is Stress Urinary Incontinence?

Stress urinary incontinence affects women of all ages including young mothers, pre-menopausal and post-menopausal women. The average age of onset is 48 years. For most, SUI is an embarrassing and bothersome condition. As a result, many women would rather:

- Restrict their social activities, like not leaving the home unless necessary
- Constantly be on a look-out for the nearest available toilet
- Bring along a change of underwear or clothing at all times
- Wear dark coloured clothing
- Wear bulky, uncomfortable pads or diapers to absorb the leakage

What Causes SUI In Women?

SUI occurs when the muscles and tissues that work to hold urine in the bladder during physical activity become weak or damaged, and are unable to keep the urethra closed when the bladder pressure suddenly increases such as when a person sneezes or coughs. This condition is caused by a weakening of the pelvic floor support (muscles and ligaments) resulting from pregnancy, childbirth, uterine prolapse and menopause. It may also be due to an inherent problem in the urethra itself.

Conditions that chronically increase pressure within the abdomen may further worsen the problem. These include obesity, chronic coughing, constipation and heavy lifting. SUI can also be worsened by oestrogen (hormonal) deficit that accompanies menopause.

What Investigations May a SUI Patient Need to Undergo?

The following tests may be required:

1. **Urine microscopy and culture test** — to diagnose urinary tract infection (UTI), as it needs to be treated aggressively before further investigations can be done.
2. **Pad test** — the patient will be asked to drink 500 ml of water. She will wear a pre-weighed sanitary pad which will be weighed one hour later. During this time, she will be asked to perform a series of activities such as walking, bending, coughing and climbing stairs. This is done to quantify her level of incontinence. Currently, this test is less frequently used due to the inconvenience caused in its implementation.
3. **Erect stress test** — the patient is asked to cough 10 times while standing on a pre-weighed absorbent sheet. The absorbent sheet will be weighed again to determine the amount of urine loss (Fig. 7.2).

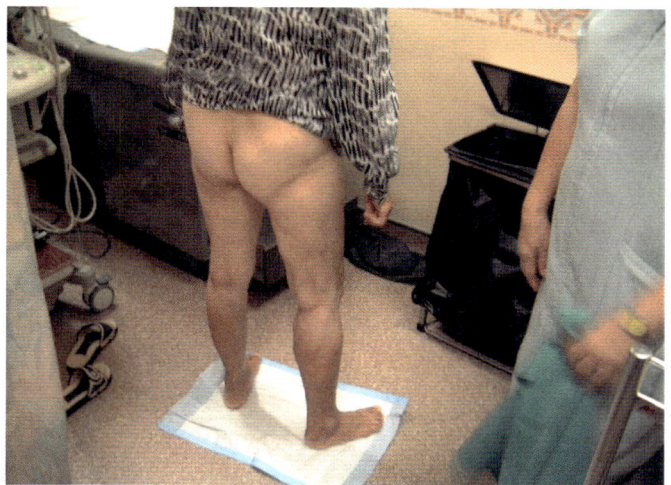

Fig. 7.2. Erect stress test — to demonstrate urine leakage.

4. **Residual urine measurement** — aids in diagnosing voiding difficulties and overflow incontinence. The measurement can be made either by performing a bladder scan or by inserting a catheter to drain the residual urine.

5. **Uroflometry** — measures the urinary flow rate to screen for voiding disorders (Fig. 7.3).

6. **Filling and voiding cystometry** — measures the pressure produced by the bladder muscles when the bladder is being filled with a sterile fluid, and during activities like coughing and passing urine. It helps in differentiating the various types of urinary incontinence and voiding disorders (Fig. 7.4).

7. **Ultrasound scan** — to exclude associated gynaecological conditions like fibroids or ovarian cysts. It is also used to measure bladder residual volumes and check bladder neck hypermobility (Fig. 7.5).

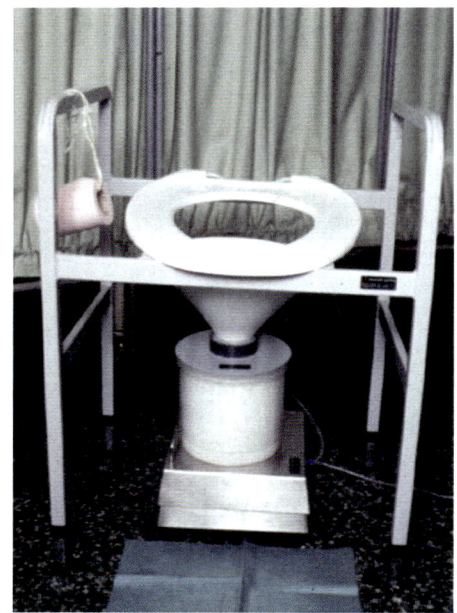

Fig. 7.3.   Uroflowmeter — to measure urinary flow rate.

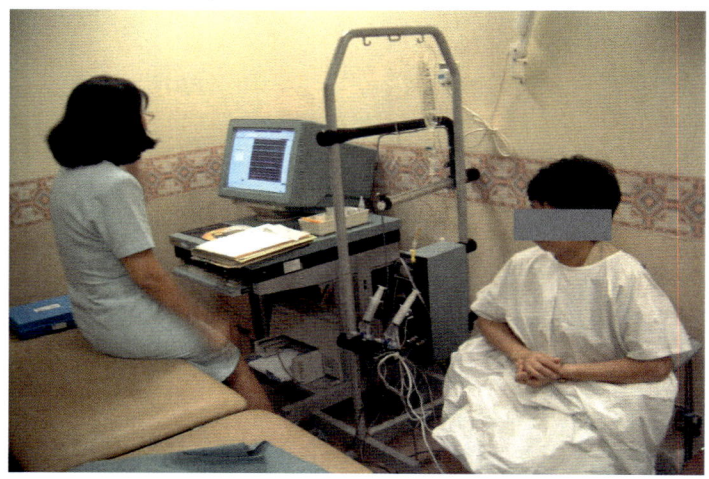

Fig. 7.4.   A patient undergoing filling and voiding cystometry.

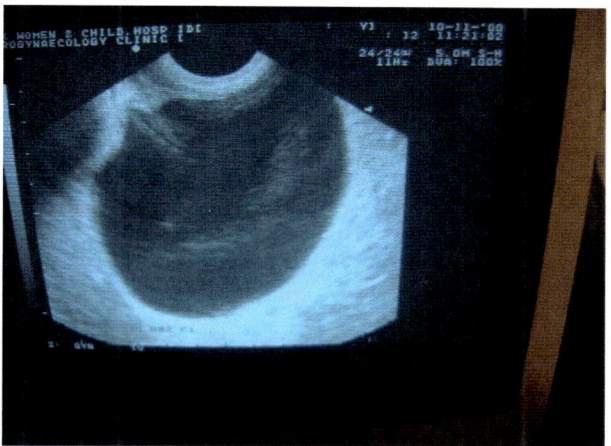

Fig. 7.5. An ultrasound image of the bladder.

Are There Any Treatments Available?

The good news is SUI is curable. While many women resort to using adult diapers or try to live with their condition, they should consider undergoing treatment. Treatments can be divided into conservative and surgical treatment. At present, there are no effective drugs for treating SUI.

Conservative treatment

1) Pelvic floor exercises (Kegel exercises)

At KK Hospital, the physiotherapist teaches patients pelvic floor exercises (PFE) to strengthen their pelvic floor muscles. These exercises will have to be done daily. At follow-up sessions, the patients' performance will be reviewed and any mistakes they might make in doing the PFE will then be corrected. For those patients whose pelvic floor muscles remain weak, adjunctive treatments for strengthening the pelvic floor muscles will be recommended.

2)   Use of vaginal cones

Vaginal cones may be used as an adjunct therapy to help patients train their pelvic floor muscles. Cones of increasing weight are used sequentially, and the patient has to retain the cone in the vagina by contracting the pelvic floor muscles. With improving muscle tone, heavier cones can be used to further improve the pelvic floor muscle tone and strength.

3)   Electrical stimulation

An electrical current is used to stimulate the pelvic floor muscles to contract. It is a second-line treatment for women who show poor results in performing pelvic floor exercises.

Improvement from the above treatment options is usually observed only after 2 to 3 months. If there is no improvement, surgical intervention should be considered.

Surgical treatment

The objective of surgery is to restore urinary continence. If the patient has an associated pelvic organ prolapse, she may be advised to undergo pelvic floor reconstructive surgery too. The main types of surgery are:

1. **Minimally invasive mid-urethral sling procedures** (Figs. 7.6 to 7.9). There are a multitude of different mid-urethral sling systems on the market, involving various different ways of inserting a tape under the urethra to achieve continence. The latest insertion techniques all purport to be safer than other previous methods. There are also a whole host of different sling materials on the market, all with different beneficial properties (according to their manufacturers). The sling system used at the KK Hospital (KKH) is the Gynecare tension-free vaginal tape (TVT) (Figs. 7.6 and 7.7) and TVT-obturator (TVT-O) (Figs. 7.8 and 7.9). This is a relatively new method and has enjoyed a very good success rate of up to 95% since the

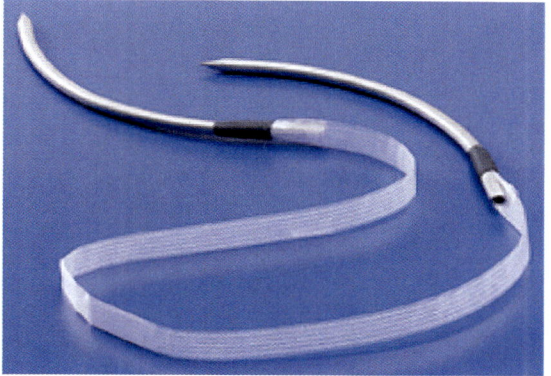

Fig. 7.6. Tension-free vaginal tape. (*Courtesy of Johnson and Johnson Medical Ltd.*)

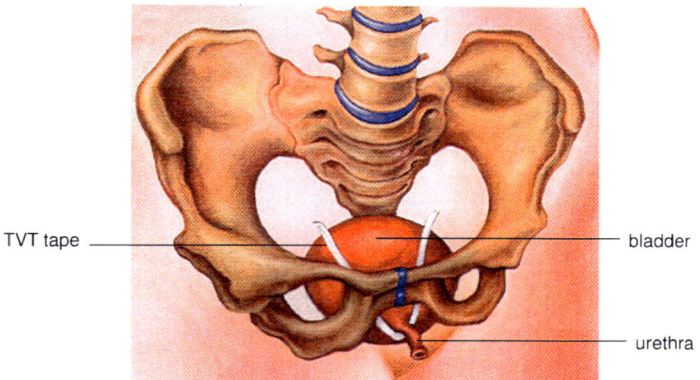

TVT tape — bladder

urethra

Fig. 7.7. TVT sling position — U-shaped support (retropubic tape). (*Courtesy of Johnson and Johnson Medical Ltd.*)

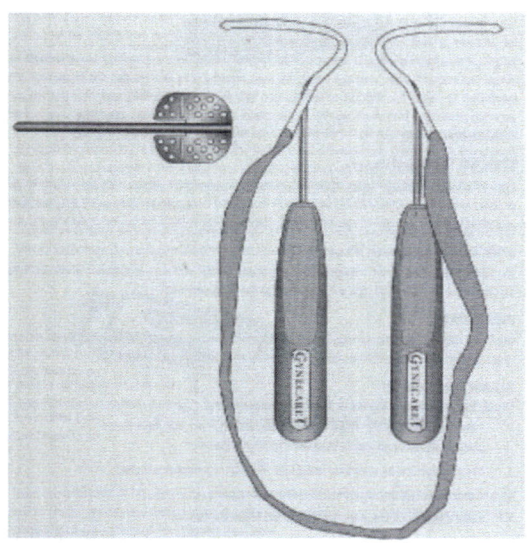

Fig. 7.8.   TVT-O Device.

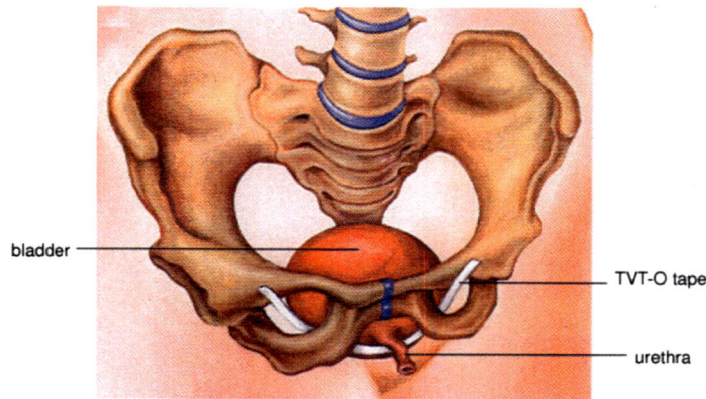

Fig. 7.9.   TVT-O sling position — hammock-shaped support (transobturator tape). (*Courtesy of Johnson and Johnson Medical Ltd.*)

KKH started using it in 1998. It has become the most common type of continence surgery performed at KKH and around the world. This procedure has the advantage that it involves less pain and can be done as a day surgery case. It has relatively minimal complications — bladder injury, bleeding, infection due to the tape, tape erosion and/or rejection — as compared with other sling systems.

2. **Burch colposuspension** — this has been superseded by the TVT/TVT-O method in recent years but is still a reliable procedure used in treating female SUI. It has an 85% success rate in the first year and up to 70% after 10 years. This surgery requires a 7 cm abdominal incision with an average of a 4-day hospital stay (Fig. 7.10).

3. Other surgeries include needle bladder neck suspension, anterior colporrhaphy with Kelly sutures, and so on. The mentioned surgeries, not performed in KKH, show lesser degrees of success than the TVT, TVT-O or the Burch colposuspension.

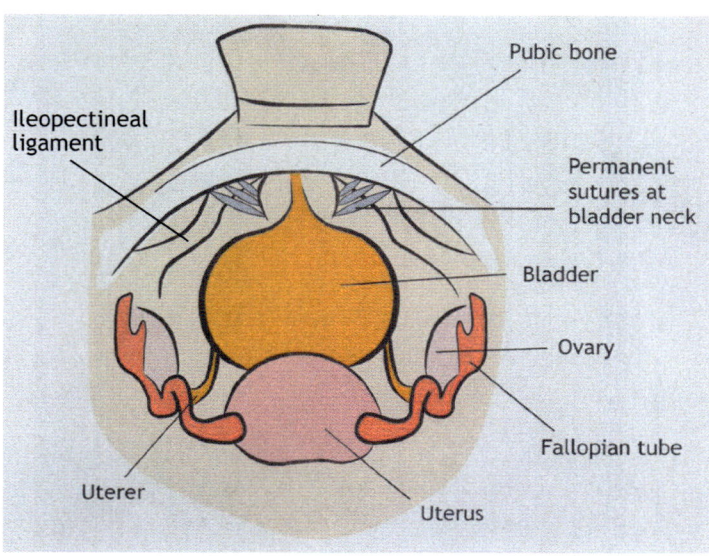

Pubic bone

Ileopectineal ligament

Permanent sutures at bladder neck

Bladder

Ovary

Fallopian tube

Uterer

Uterus

Fig. 7.10. Burch colposuspension — permanent sutures placed at bladder neck to achieve urinary continence.

Myths About Stress Urinary Incontinence

Myth #1: SUI is a part of the "natural" ageing process from which one cannot escape.

False. SUI is not a natural or normal condition as the supporting structures around the urethra fail to function properly for various reasons. People usually adjust their daily activities to hide this embarrassing condition. There may come a time when these people are unable to engage in these activities, adversely affecting their quality of life. Seeking the help of a doctor is necessary to solve the problem.

Myth #2: It's too late for older women to be treated for stress urinary incontinence.

False. One is never too young or old to start treatment. It is never too late to improve one's quality of life. In fact, many patients with SUI see an improvement and are happier after treatment.

Myth #3: Young women do not need to worry about SUI because only "old ladies" get it.

False. Although most females who suffer from this condition are post-menopausal women, about one third of women with SUI begin showing symptoms before the age of 35.

Myth #4: Practising pelvic floor exercises will totally prevent bladder problems.

False. Pelvic floor exercises may be effective (dependent on how conscientiously they are performed) in improving SUI for some women, but they are not effective for all women.

Myth #5: After surgery, SUI never recurs and as such, there is no need for any follow-up.

False. There is a small but definitive failure rate. This can be minimised by having an experienced surgeon (urogynaecologist) perform the surgery. Postoperatively, the patient should carry only light loads, avoid constipation, and avoid pregnancy as vaginal delivery may nullify the benefits of continence surgery. Lastly, as the tape is a foreign body, it is necessary that the patient goes for regular check-ups to ensure there is no problem with the tape.

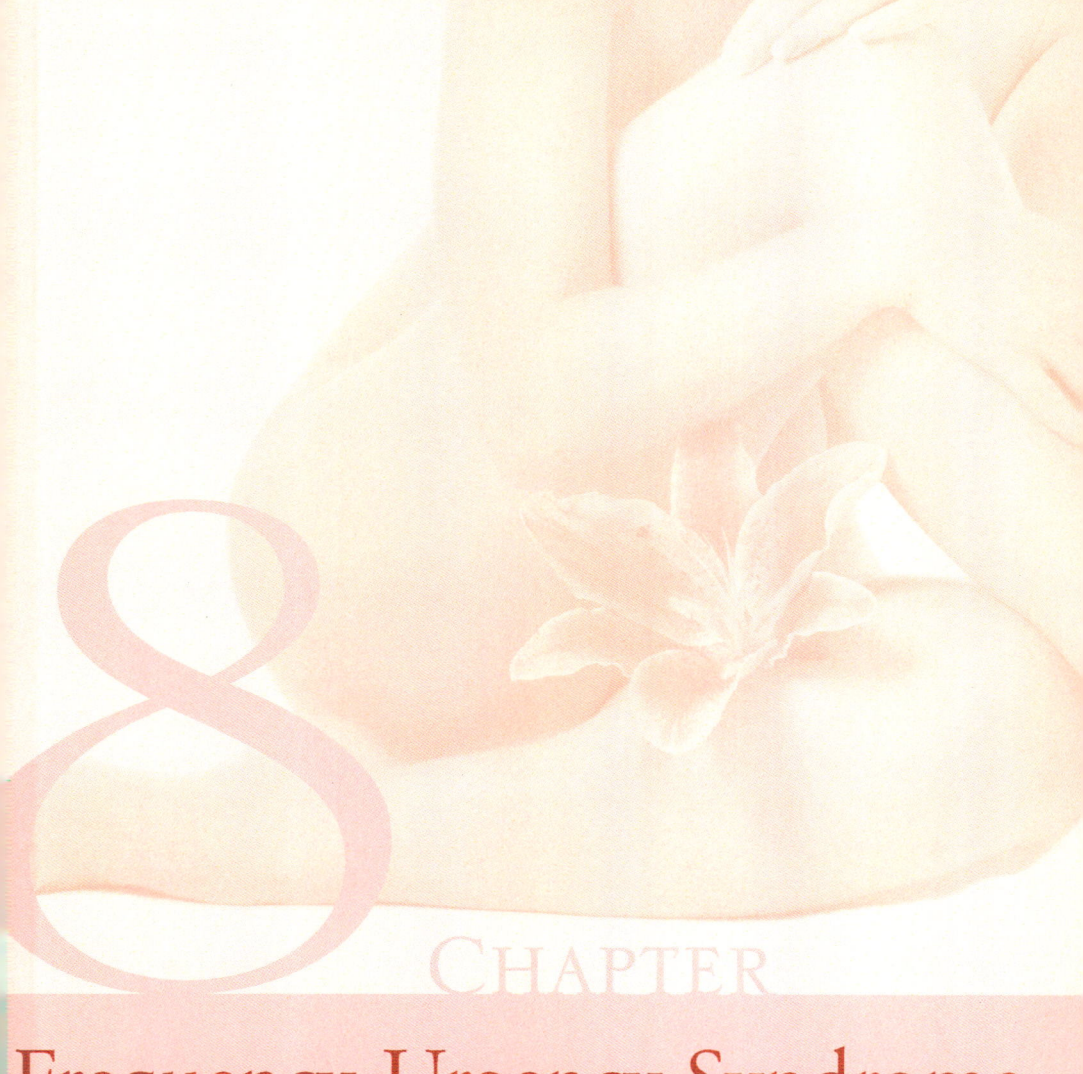

8
CHAPTER

Frequency-Urgency Syndrome
or the
Overactive Bladder Syndrome

"Doctor, why am I always going to the toilet to pass urine?"

Introduction

Apart from stress urinary incontinence (SUI), there is another type of urinary incontinence, in which the sensation of needing to urinate is overwhelming and difficult to defer. It is called urgency urinary incontinence (UUI) and is associated with frequency-urgency syndrome (FUS), which is more commonly known as overactive bladder syndrome (OAB).

Overactive bladder syndrome occurs in 40% of people with urinary leakage, and is the second most common cause of incontinence. About 10% of the general population suffer from this condition, which tends to occur more often with age. OAB is also more common in menopausal women and especially those who have spinal cord injuries, pelvic surgery, diseases like diabetes mellitus, multiple sclerosis, or radiation treatment for the pelvis. Idiopathic OAB, where there is no identifiable cause, is the most common type.

Symptoms of OAB/FUS

This problem is usually present when a person:

1. Has a sudden, overwhelming need to urinate (urgency) (Fig. 8.1)
2. Has to urinate more than 7 times during the day (frequency)

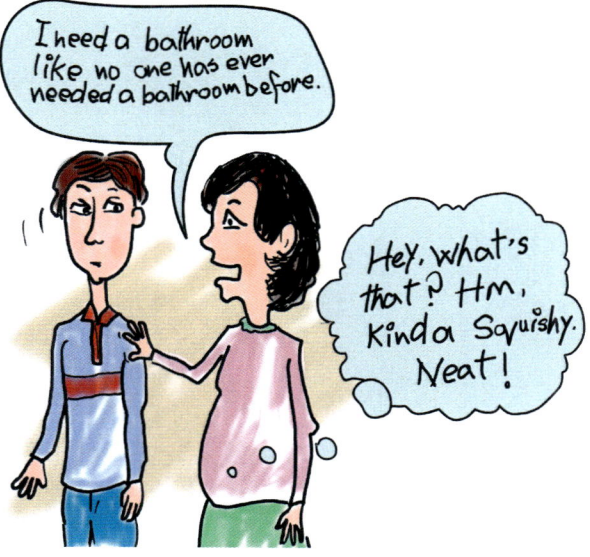

Fig. 8.1. Pregnancy-associated urgency.

3. Wakes up more than once in the night to urinate (nocturia) (Fig. 8.2)

4. Suffers from leakage of urine before she could reach the toilet.

Occasionally, UUI occurs during sexual intercourse, especially during orgasm or sexual climax. This can adversely affect a couple's sex life and result in severe embarrassment and a loss of self-worth (Fig. 8.3).

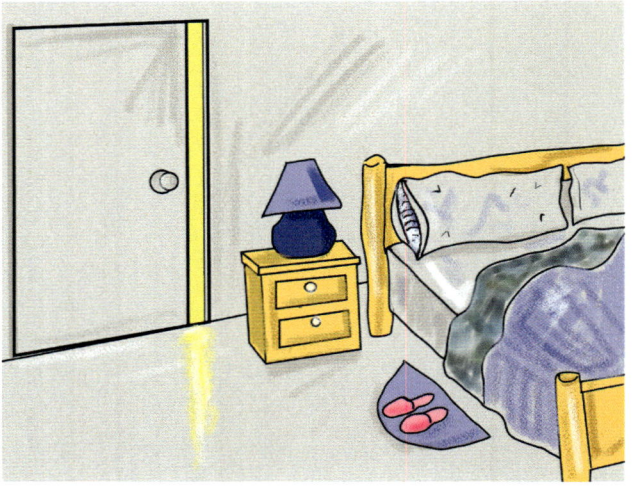

Fig. 8.2. Disruption of sleep due to nocturia.

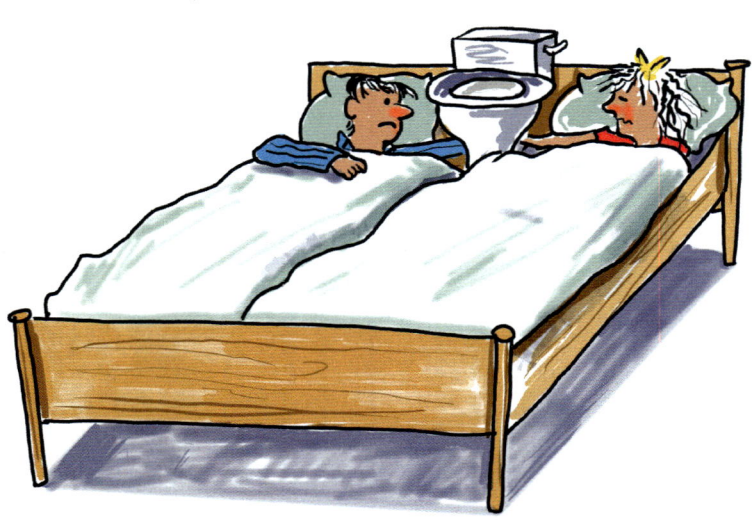

Fig. 8.3. OAB affecting intimacy, causing embarrassment and lack of self-worth.

Common Causes of OAB/FUS

The bladder's main function is to store and release urine. In general, the human body produces 1 mL of urine per minute throughout the day. Women develop symptoms of frequency, urgency, nocturia and possibly incontinence if their bladders are:

- relatively inextensible
- hypersensitive to stimulation
- prone to abnormal contractions

As mentioned previously, idiopathic OAB, where there is no identifiable cause, is the most common type of OAB. However, other identifiable causes of OAB symptoms should be determined and the patient treated first, before such a diagnosis is made.

1. Urinary tract infection (UTI). This is one of the most common causes of OAB symptoms and should be treated before further investigations are carried out to diagnose OAB (Fig. 8.4).
2. Pelvic organ prolapse (POP). This can also cause OAB symptoms because of obstruction of the urethra (Fig. 8.5). Treatment involves surgery or a ring pessary.
3. Urogenital atrophy, which occurs due to lack of oestrogen in menopausal women, can give rise to OAB symptoms. The problem can be treated with the use of topical oestrogen cream, pessaries or hormone impregnated ring pessaries.
4. Tumorous growths in the female reproductive tract, like fibroids (Fig. 8.6) and ovarian cysts or masses (Fig. 8.7), can exert pressure on the bladder, causing OAB symptoms. Surgical removal of such growths is necessary to bring about relief.
5. Common medical conditions like constipation (Fig. 8.8), diabetes mellitus, and congestive cardiac failure all

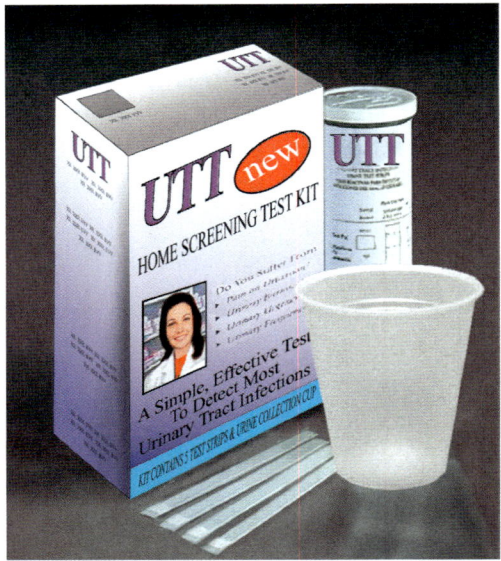

Fig. 8.4.   Urinary   tract   infection   —   needs   to   be   treated aggressively and excluded before further investigations for OAB can be done.

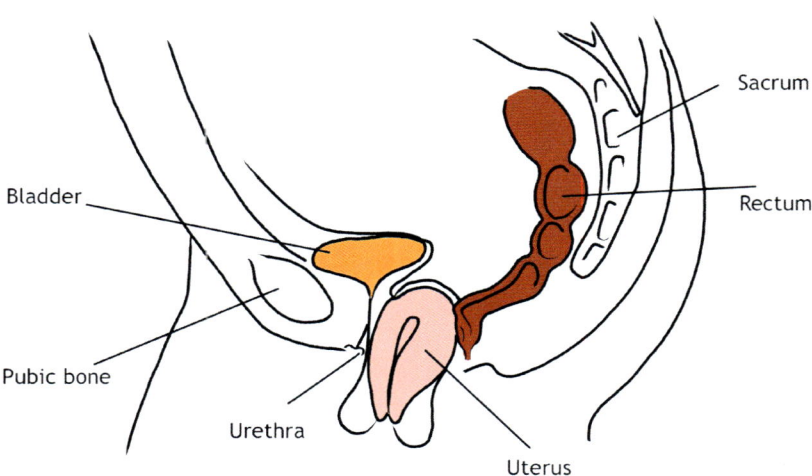

Fig. 8.5.   Pelvic organ prolapse.

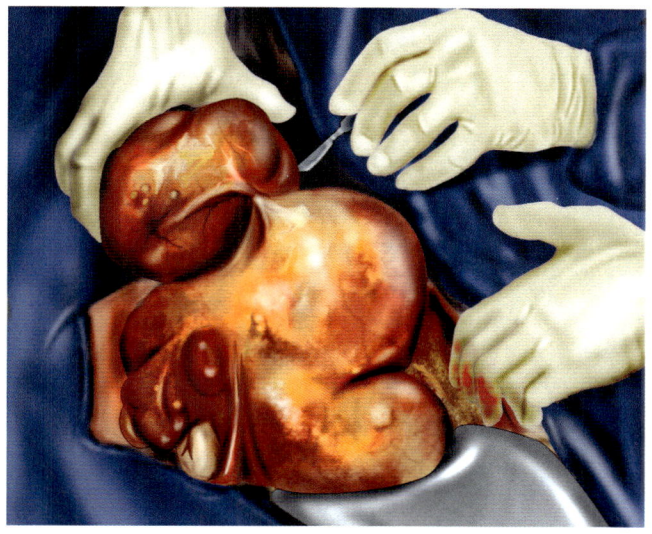

Fig. 8.6.   Uterus with multiple fibroids at surgery.

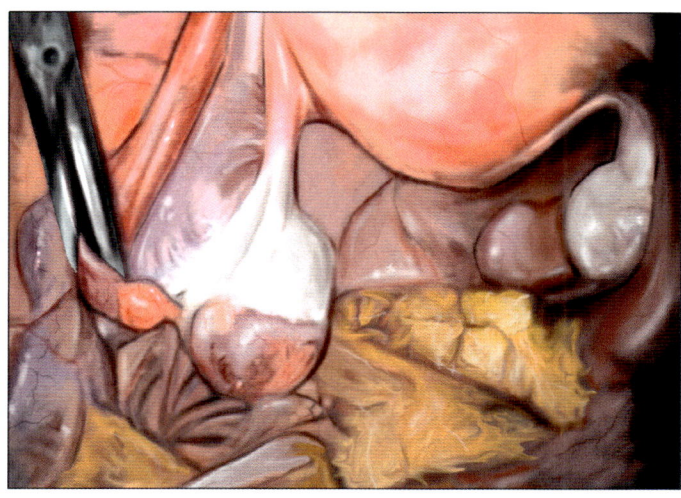

Fig. 8.7.   Ovarian cyst of left ovary.

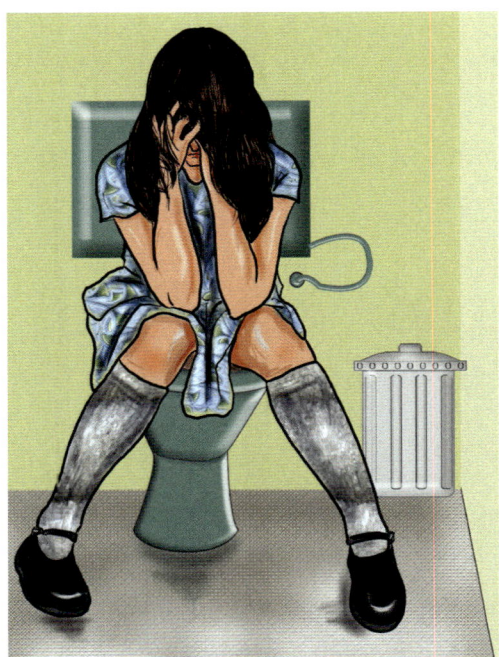

Fig. 8.8.   Constipation.

contribute to the worsening of OAB symptoms. However, certain medications themselves can cause OAB symptoms, such as diuretics (used in the treatment of hypertension or heart failure) and certain psychiatric medications (Fig. 8.9).

6.   Previous pelvic surgery or radiation therapy for certain gynaecological cancers, can cause OAB symptoms. Radiation treatment can also contribute to the risk of getting bladder cancer (Fig. 8.10), and this presents with severe OAB symptoms, as well as blood in the urine (haematuria). Bladder cancer needs urgent referral to the urology specialists, as do bladder stones (calculi), for definitive treatment.

7. Certain psychological problems like general anxiety and fear can result in worsening of OAB symptoms, as well as the psychological fear of urinary leakage and associated embarrassment. This can lead to certain bad habits like over-frequent toileting, which reinforces a vicious cycle of frequency and urgency. Other bad habits include excessive intake of fluids, and overuse of caffeinated beverages or alcohol, leading to a worsening pattern of OAB.

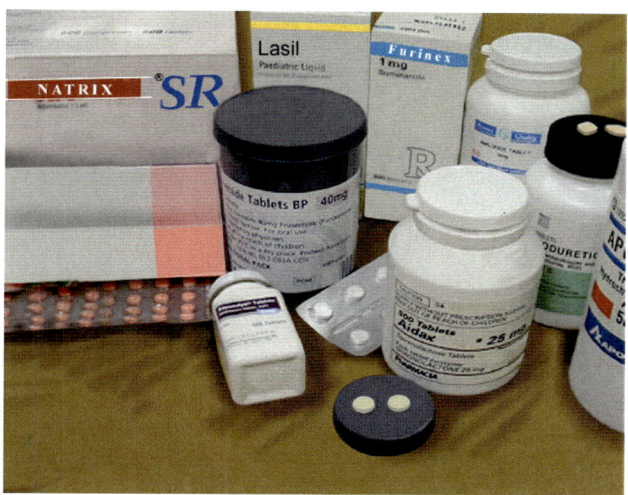

Fig. 8.9. Diuretics and other medications.

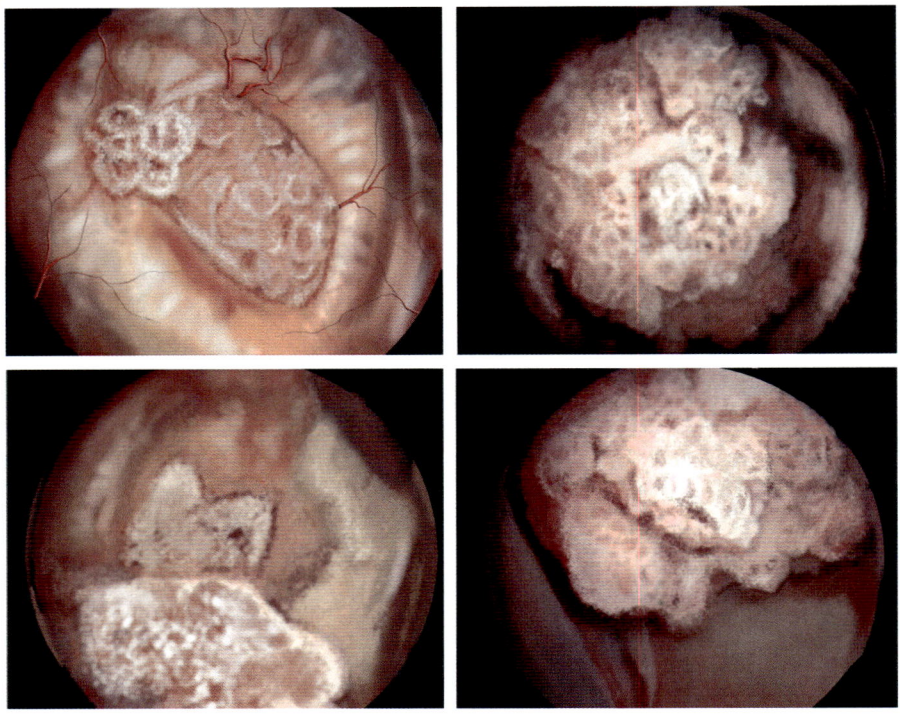

Fig. 8.10.   Bladder cancer — visualised during cystoscopy.

This is by no means a comprehensive list of causes of FUS/OAB. It provides a description of some of the more common causes and an idea of how doctors manage the problems.

Investigations

Simple tests include:

- Urine microscopy and urine culture — to rule out UTI.
- Bladder diary — to assess drinking habits, frequency of urination, volume and timing of fluid intake and urine discharged, and episodes of urine leakage.
- Pad testing — as a means of diagnosing incontinence and a semi-quantitative assessment of severity.
- Uroflowmetry — to assess ease of passing urine by measuring the urine flow rate.

Complex tests include:

- Cystometry and urethral pressure profilometry (UPP)
- Ultrasound pelvis and ultrasound kidneys/bladder
- Cystoscopy
- Videourodynamic study
- Ambulatory urodynamics

For a more thorough description of the complex investigations, please refer to Chapter 4. Only in rare cases will videourodynamic studies or ambulatory urodynamic studies be performed — this is usually done for complex cases in which all other previous treatments were unsuccessful.

Management of OAB/FUS

Many patients think that surgery is the ultimate cure for all forms of urinary leakage. But this could not be further from the truth. It is important to find out what type of urinary incontinence the patient has, as this will determine the type of treatment required.

For OAB/FUS sufferers, surgery is the final resort, only after all other medical options have failed to control a patient's urinary symptoms.

Conservative treatment

Non-medical treatment

The non-medical modalities include the following:

1) Incorporating lifestyle changes like reducing fluid intake can help patients, especially those who over-drink.
2) Reducing intake of beverages that contain caffeine such as coffee and tea (caffeine is a diuretic and a bladder irritant).
3) Cutting down on alcohol consumption (as alcohol is a diuretic and bladder irritant).
4) Embarking on a controlled weight-loss programme with exercise and a sensible diet, as OAB/FUS symptoms can be caused by obesity.
5) Managing other medical problems like diabetes mellitus, whereby diet control, oral medication or insulin treatment will help improve urinary symptoms.
6) Stop medications like diuretics (for treatment of heart failure), which can worsen incontinence symptoms, or certain medications for psychiatric treatment (as these can also give rise to urinary symptoms). However, the patients need to consult with their respective doctors before stopping these medications.
7) Undergoing physiotherapy such as pelvic floor exercises (PFE) and bladder retraining methods, under the guidance of a physiotherapist, to improve urinary control.
   — PFE involves squeezing the layer of muscles (levator ani muscles), that support the urethra, the vagina and rectum. By mastering PFE, its daily practice will bring about reduced urinary leakage over time.
   — bladder retraining methods include bladder drill, biofeedback and electrical (faradic) stimulation, and are carried out under the guidance of a physiotherapist.

These can be done in conjunction with PFE with the aim of improving bladder control and reducing urinary leakage.

— the advantages of physiotherapy is that the use of drugs and medications, which have side effects, can be avoided. Unfortunately, the benefits wear off once a patient stops PFE.

Medical treatment

Currently, treatment for OAB/FUS involves mostly the use of medications, the most commonly used being anti-muscarinic agents. They act by:

1) Allowing the bladder to relax and stretch
2) Allowing more urine to accumulate in the bladder before the patient feels the urge to urinate
3) Stopping unwanted bladder contractions

Oxybutynin and tolterodine are the common anti-muscarinic medications prescribed to treat OAB/FUS presently available at the KK Hospital.

Unfortunately, as with all medications, there are side effects which patients may find them difficult to tolerate. The most common side effects include:

- Dry mouth (Fig. 8.11)
- Constipation
- Blurring of vision
- Drowsiness

Different medications are efficacious in different individuals. This issue of finding a suitable medication with minimal side effects is best discussed with a doctor or urogynaecologist, who may recommend a trial of anti-muscarinic medication.

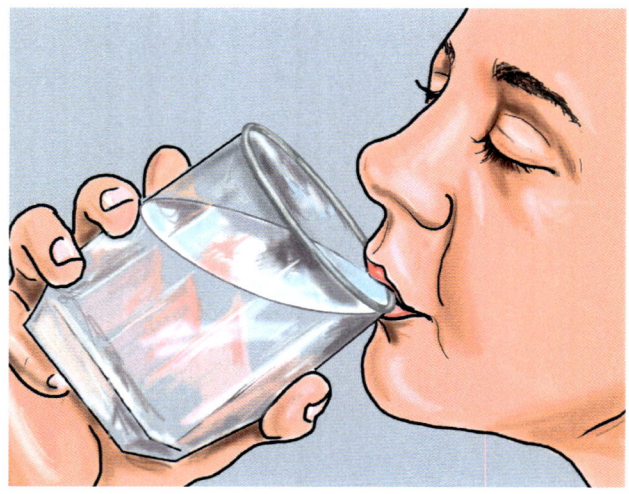

Fig. 8.11.   Dry mouth secondary to anti-muscarinic drugs — the wrong thing to do is to drink more to relieve dry mouth as urinary symptoms can worsen.

There are other medications that help patients with FUS/OAB. These include imipramine and desmopressin. Imipramine is useful for treating nocturnal symptoms (nocturia). Desmopressin is used specifically to alleviate nocturnal urinary symptoms, and works by reducing the kidney's urine production. Desmopressin can be used in elderly patients, but it occasionally causes low salt levels (hyponatraemia) in the patient's blood, and a kidney function blood test is required if an elderly patient is started on it.

Surgical treatment

Details of many different types of surgical operations — tried and tested on patients with severe OAB/FUS — can be found in textbooks. Some methods involve attaching a piece of small intestine to the bladder to increase the bladder capacity and reduce abnormal contractions. Other forms of surgery involve a diversion of the ureters away from the bladder into a segment of the small intestine, that comes through the patient's abdominal wall. For hygiene reasons and to minimise skin damage the patient would require a plastic bag (stoma bag) to be attached to her abdomen for urine collection.

Surgery is usually the last resort due to various reasons, which include relatively high complication rates, possible disfigurement, limited success rates, as well as the potential for serious health problems in the long run, such as cancer developing in the small bowel segments used in such operations.

Conclusion

OAB/FUS is a chronic and frustrating condition faced by many women. There are, however, many sensible lifestyle changes and habits which they can adopt to prevent or control OAB symptoms.

The use of physiotherapy has seen good results in symptom control and can be a viable long-term option to manage OAB/FUS. Medication is very useful for acute symptom control but has some unwanted side effects. However, these detrimental effects may be minimised or avoided with the prescription of suitable drugs by a specialist doctor.

When someone is troubled by FUS/OAB, she should not ignore it. Instead she should seek the help of her doctor.

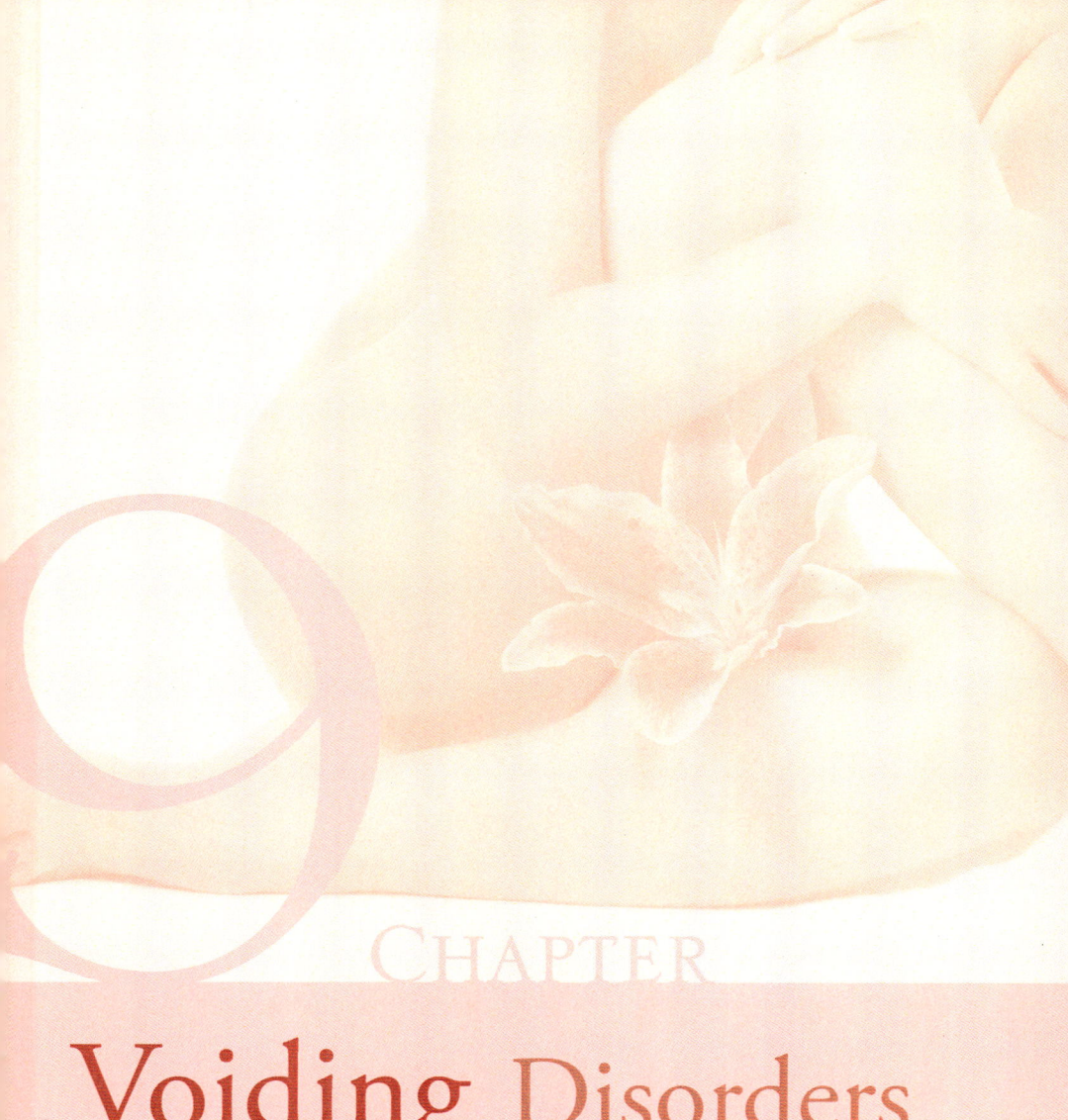

CHAPTER

9

Voiding Disorders

"Doctor, why is my urine stream so slow?"

What is Voiding Disorder?

Voiding disorders develop when a patient has difficulty emptying her bladder of urine. This may be due to the bladder failing to contract (detrusor failure), or an outflow obstruction in the urine tube (urethra), or a combination of both.

Symptoms ranging from difficulty in starting urine flow (hesitancy) to acute or chronic urinary retention may be present in patients.

Voiding disorders are surprisingly common, occurring in up to 14% of women with urinary problems. In some cases, voiding disorders can develop alongside stress urinary incontinence (see Chapter 7) and overactive bladder syndrome (see Chapter 8).

Definitions

Acute retention of urine (ARU) i.e. the sudden inability to urinate, is usually painful. There are occasions in which ARU may not be painful, as in the case of epidural anaesthesia or a slipped disc.

Chronic retention of urine is usually not painful. The patient may also suffer from overflow incontinence with chronic retention of urine, and there is a grossly distended bladder on examination.

Causes of Voiding Disorders In Women

Medication-related causes

- Epidural anaesthesia — one of the commonest causes
- Anticholinergic drugs — used in OAB treatment

Obstructive causes

Conditions arising from obstructive causes are more common in men (due to enlargement of the prostate gland) but can still occur in women. The causes include:

- Previous continence surgery
- Severe pelvic organ prolapse (approximately 50% of cases)
- Urethral stricture due to chronic inflammation, or atrophy due to menopause (13% of cases)
- External pressure from a posterior uterine fibroid or compression from other pelvic masses
- Faecal impaction from constipation
- Foreign bodies
- Bladder stones

Inflammatory causes

Conditions causing pain in the abdomen, vagina or urethra can cause urinary retention. These include:

- Postoperative pain
- Chemical or allergic irritants
- Active vulval herpes infection

Bladder failure

When the bladder becomes large and flaccid, with little or no muscle tone or function, overflow incontinence occurs. The sequelae of this include:

- Reduced functional ability of the bladder to expel urine efficiently
- Frequent urination i.e. the symptom of frequency
- Recurrent urinary tract infection (RUTI)
- Hydroureter and hydronephrosis, where there is physical damage and swelling of the ureters and kidneys due to backflow of urine
- Chronic renal failure

Fowler's syndrome

Some women develop ARU or some degree of voiding dysfunction, due to the failure of the urethral sphincter (the urethral muscle that keeps a person continent) to relax. This prevents urine from being passed normally when the bladder contracts to expel urine.

Spinal problems

The cauda equina syndrome is a spinal cord condition due to compression by a slipped disc, causing low back pain, leg weakness, sensory loss in the buttock area, voiding difficulty, or even urinary incontinence. This condition is a surgical emergency, and must be attended to by an orthopaedic surgeon.

Multiple sclerosis

Multiple sclerosis is a rare nerve disorder, occurring more commonly in Caucasians. It usually presents with symptoms of urgency, frequency and urge incontinence, although it can also cause voiding difficulties and incomplete bladder emptying. This is an unusual disease as the pattern of symptoms changes with each episode, making its diagnosis and management difficult. Fortunately, it is rare in Southeast Asia.

Clinical Features

Women are rarely asymptomatic. Most with voiding difficulty present with:

- Poor urine stream
- Increased episodes of urination
- A feeling of incomplete emptying
- Straining to urinate
- Prolonged duration of urination to empty bladder
- Overflow incontinence
- Pain due to an acutely over distended bladder

Investigations

1. Frequency-volume chart/bladder diary

— Frequent micturition of small volumes with incontinence suggest overflow.

2. Bedside bladder scan (Fig. 9.1)

— The patient should be asked to void before the ultrasound scan is performed.
— A post-void residual volume of more than 50 ml is not normal (Fig. 9.2).

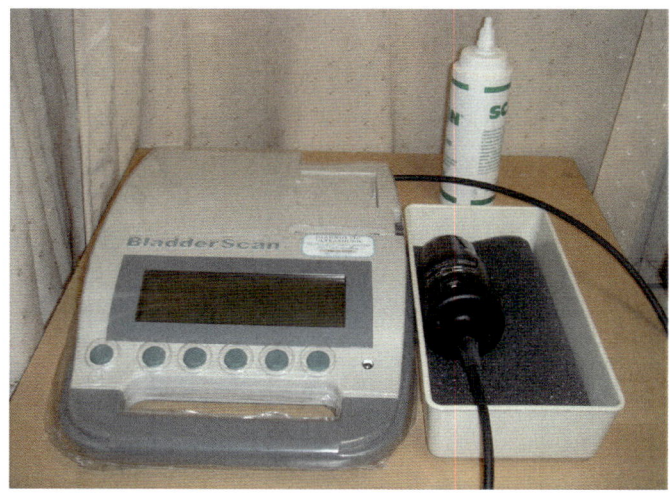

Fig. 9.1.   A bladder scanner.

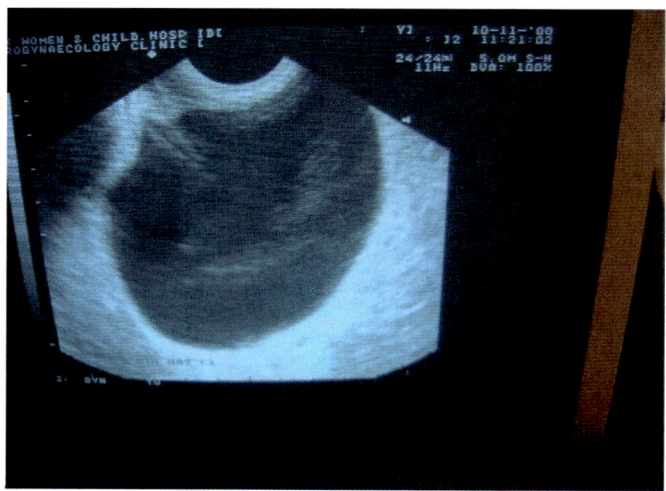

Fig. 9.2.   Overfull bladder as seen via transvaginal ultrasound.

3. Uroflowmetry

— The patient should sit normally on the commode, with repeat measurements being taken in full privacy.
— Repeated flow rates of less than 15 ml/sec, when the voided volume is more than 150 ml, suggest voiding difficulty.

4. Cystometry

— This form of urodynamic testing will differentiate between urethral outflow obstruction (high bladder pressure and low urine flow) and bladder muscle (detrusor) failure (low bladder pressure and low urine flow).

5. Urethral pressure profilometry

— This test is useful for identifying a possible urethral obstruction.

6. Radiographic imaging includes:

— Pelvic ultrasound to look for pelvic masses like a large uterine fibroid
— Renal ultrasound scan or an IVU (intravenous urogram) to assess the kidneys, ureters and bladder
— CT (computerised tomography) or MRI (magnetic resonance imaging) to assess pelvic masses or spinal cord lesions which may cause obstructive urinary symptoms.

Treatment

1. Behavioural modification

- Suprapubic pressure during urination to aid in emptying the bladder
- Anticholinergic drugs should be stopped
- Double voiding to remove chronic residual urine so as to prevent urinary tract infection (UTI) and frequent urination

In cases of mild voiding difficulty following continence surgery, a change to a more reclined posture when seated on the toilet seat during urination may help ease urine flow.

2. Medical treatment

- There are medications that can be prescribed to improve bladder muscle contraction and urethral muscle relaxation so as to enable urine to be easily passed.
- The efficacy of such medications is very variable and the degree of benefit may be small. Also, because of the side effects that arise, such medications have limited long term use.

3. Catheterisation

- In ARU, the bladder should be decompressed and allowed to rest for a day or more by having an indwelling catheter inserted (Fig. 9.3).
- A period of bladder retraining by slowly weaning off the indwelling catheter usually helps in restoring bladder function fully.

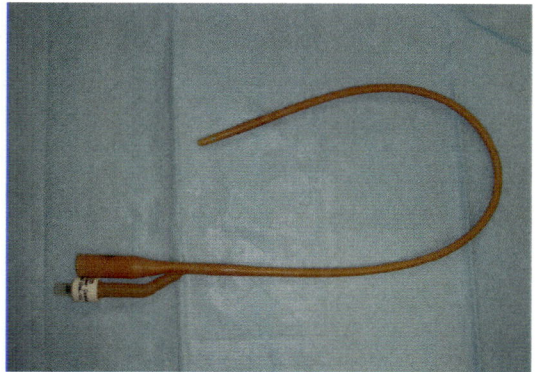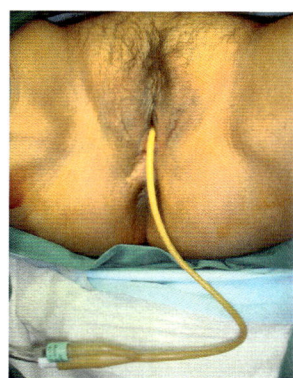

Fig. 9.3. Indwelling urethral catheter.

- Clean intermittent self-catheterisation (CISC) can be taught to women with chronic voiding difficulty, as it has a lower risk of UTI than long-term indwelling catheterisation (Fig. 9.4).
- The number of times CISC is performed each day is based on the residual volumes — when the residual urine volume is consistently less than 100–150 ml, CISC can be stopped.

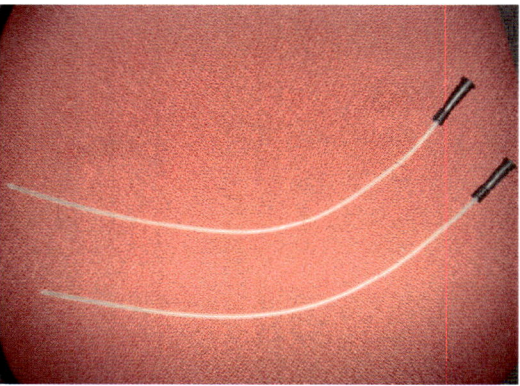

Fig. 9.4.   CISC catheters.

4. Surgery

- If a fibroid uterus or a large ovarian cyst is found to be the cause of voiding difficulty, surgical removal is required.
- If a urethral stricture is present, an operation called an Otis urethrotomy (where the stricture is released) can be done. A large diameter catheter is left in the body for two weeks to allow for healing, and CISC on a weekly basis is used to maintain patency.

Conclusion

Voiding disorders are difficult and frustrating problems faced by some women. Ignoring these problems could result in recurrent UTI, long-term bladder damage, and even kidney damage. Thankfully, there are different methods, both conservative and surgical, to control voiding difficulty.

If voiding disorder is suspected, it is important that an appointment be made with a doctor, a gynaecologist or a urogynaecologist for a comprehensive assessment and holistic management of the condition.

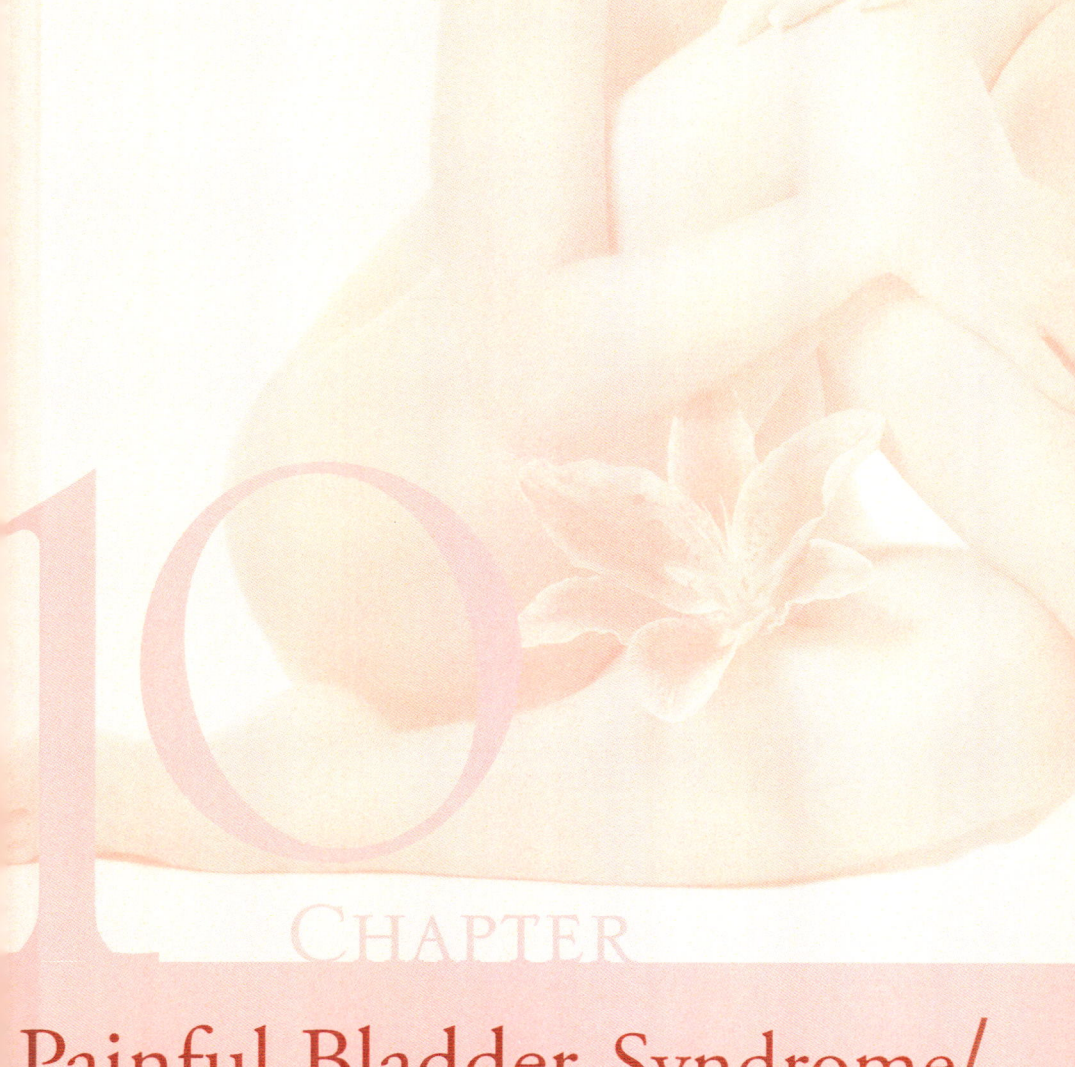

CHAPTER 10

Painful Bladder Syndrome/
Interstitial Cystitis

"Doctor, what's wrong with me? I need to pee every few minutes during the day and night."

Many women suffer from urinary frequency and urgency due to various causes. However, there is a specific bladder condition that can cause extreme urgency associated with pain, requiring the person to urinate many times during the day and night, without the presence of infection or other bladder pathology. This is called the painful bladder syndrome (PBS) or interstitial cystitis (IC).

What are the Symptoms?

Most patients complain of the need to pass urine very often during the day and night. They may feel pain in various parts of their body: lower abdomen, in the region above the pubis, the perineum, lower back, vulva and vagina in women; and in men, the pain can be localised in the penis, testes, scrotum and even the rectum.

What is Interstitial Cystitis?

The term "interstitial cystitis" (IC) was coined by Skene in 1887 to describe a chronic debilitating bladder disorder, i.e. a recurring discomfort or pain in the bladder, and the surrounding pelvic region.

In 1987, the research description of IC was proposed by the National Institute for Arthritis, Diabetes, Digestive and

Kidney Diseases (NIDDK) in the United States. This was later revised in 1988.

What is Painful Bladder Syndrome?

Painful bladder syndrome is defined by the International Continence Society in 2002 as a complaint of suprapubic pain related to bladder filling, accompanied by other symptoms such as increased daytime and night-time urinary frequency, in the absence of proven urinary infection or other obvious pathology.

PBS is the medical term that is currently used in preference to IC in patients with severe urinary frequency and urgency.

How Common is PBS?

The condition is more common in women than men (female: male = 9:1). The average age of patients is between 42 and 53 years. The incidence is between 16 and 450 per 100,000 people.

What Causes PBS?

There are many theories for what causes PBS, and why certain individuals are predisposed.

- Glycosaminoglycan (GAG) layer deficiency
- Local bladder wall disorder/systemic disease
- Mast cell degranulation
- Neurogenic inflammation
- Infection
- Autoimmune disorder
- Hypoxia/urotoxins

A detailed examination of the urothelium (surface lining of the bladder) and the protective GAG layer demonstrates that:

- The main components of an intact GAG layer are chondriotin sulphate, as well as heparin and hyaluronic acid.
- In patients with PBS, there is a reduction or lack of GAG and a significant chondriotin sulphate deficit in the urine, the GAG layer and the suburothelial bladder tissue.
- Permeability disorders of various noxious substances occur when the GAG layer is deficient. These are detected by using ultrastructural, biochemical and functional methods.

Today, medical experts agree that:

- The protective GAG layer in most PBS patients is inadequately developed and/or dysfunctional, leading to an increase in permeability (Fig. 10.1).
- GAG layer defects provide the best substantiated hypothesis for the development and progression of PBS (Fig. 10.2).
- Noxious substances trigger a cascade of inflammation and nerve-related signals that give rise to symptoms and signs (Fig. 10.3) that eventually result in a chronically scarred and contracted bladder, with severe pain and irritating urinary symptoms.

Diagnosis

Investigations are needed to exclude urinary tract and pelvic pathology such as infection or tumours which could cause similar symptoms. Urine microscopy and culture/sensitivity are necessary. Ultrasound of the pelvis/urinary tract and cystoscopy (endoscopic examination of the bladder) may be required in some patients.

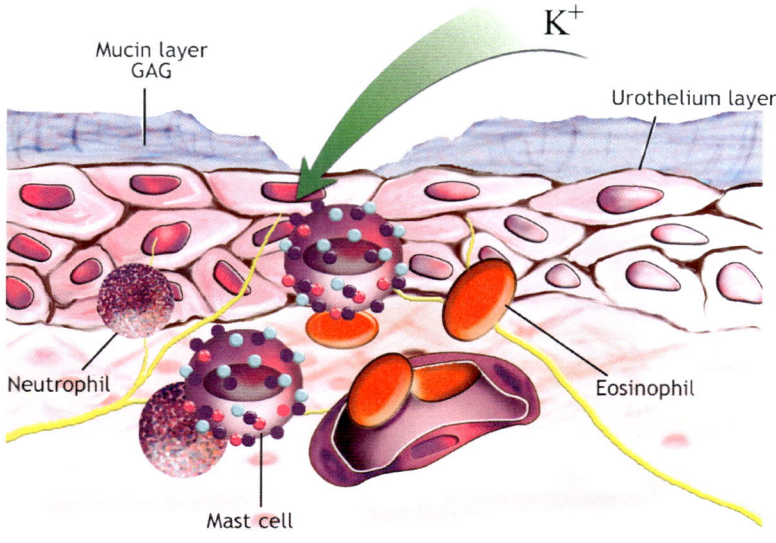

Fig. 10.1. Deficient GAG layer — allowing noxious stimuli to penetrate.

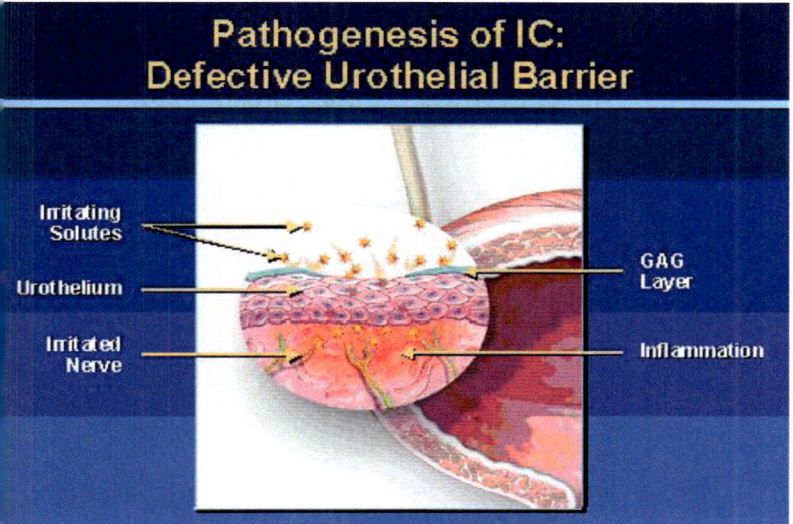

Fig. 10.2. Noxious stimuli trigger inflammatory and nerve-mediated changes, giving rise to symptoms.

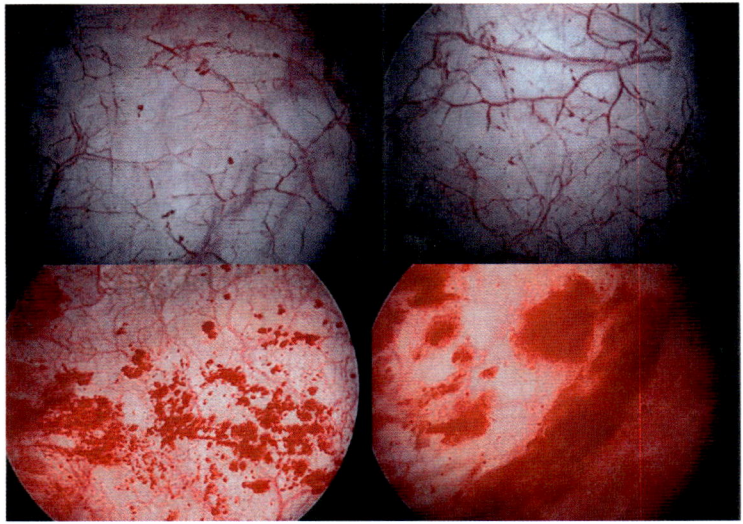

Fig. 10.3.   Cystoscopic pictures showing bladder mucosal bleeding in a PBS patient.

Management Options in PBS

There are many therapies for this condition. Treatment should be individualised.

1. **Diet.** Research on the effect of diet on PBS is limited. Some foods appear to irritate the bladder. Patients may find that avoiding these foodstuffs decrease their flare-ups. However, there appears to be great individual variation. Common food/drinks related to flare ups include:

   - Coffee, tea, soda, alcohol, citrus fruit drinks
   - Food and drinks with artificial sweeteners such as aspartame and saccharin
   - Spicy food
   - Food with high potassium content such as bananas and avocados.

2. **Oral Therapy.** Antihistamines, painkillers may be used. GAG agents such as Elmiron may help in 50–60% of patients.

3. **Intravesical Therapy** (direct instillation of medication into the bladder). Various agents such as heparin, lidocaine or dimethyl sulphoside (DMSO) had been used with variable success.

4. **Surgery.** Surgery is the last option as it has side effects and success rates are dismal.

5. **Research.** Use of botulinum toxin in the treatment of PBS shows some improvement in symptoms but this is still in the research phase.

Treatment Objectives in PBS

As the underlying cause of PBS is unclear, treatment is difficult and frequently unsatisfactory. The treatment objectives for PBS are as follows:

- Re-establish the GAG layer
- Reduce the severity of urgency
- Reduce the frequency of urination
- Increase the volume of urine passed
- Increase the bladder capacity to hold urine
- Pain relief
- Improve the patient's quality of life
- Treat concomitant diseases.

Conservative treatment includes delivering various chemicals and drugs directly into the bladder to replace or replenish the GAG layer such as chondroitin sulphate, hyaluronic acid, heparin, dimethyl sulfoxide (DMSO), or a combination of all of the above. The success rates range from 30% to 92%.

Oral medication such as painkillers, antihistamines, antidepressants, polypentosan polysulfate or a combination of treatments have been used. However, there is no conclusive evidence for the success of this mode of treatment.

Some patients have worsening urinary frequency and urgency after consuming certain foods (usually acidic foods such as oranges, tomatoes, etc.). By avoiding these foods, one may be able to reduce the symptoms of PBS.

Surgery for PBS is associated with low success but a high complication rate. Hence, it is not commonly practised or advocated.

To date, only two drugs — DMSO and polypentosan polysulfate — have been approved by the US Food & Drug Administration (FDA) for use in the United States to treat PBS.

Conclusion

1. PBS/IC can have multiple causes, without any clear underlying cause confirmed as yet.
2. A variety of empirical treatments have been used. No single treatment works for all patients.
3. The best approach is with sequential treatment trials, starting with the least toxic choices, until a satisfactory level of relief is achieved.
4. PBS/IC is a difficult condition to endure and patients will cope best with supportive and understanding friends, relatives, and medical and nursing practitioners.

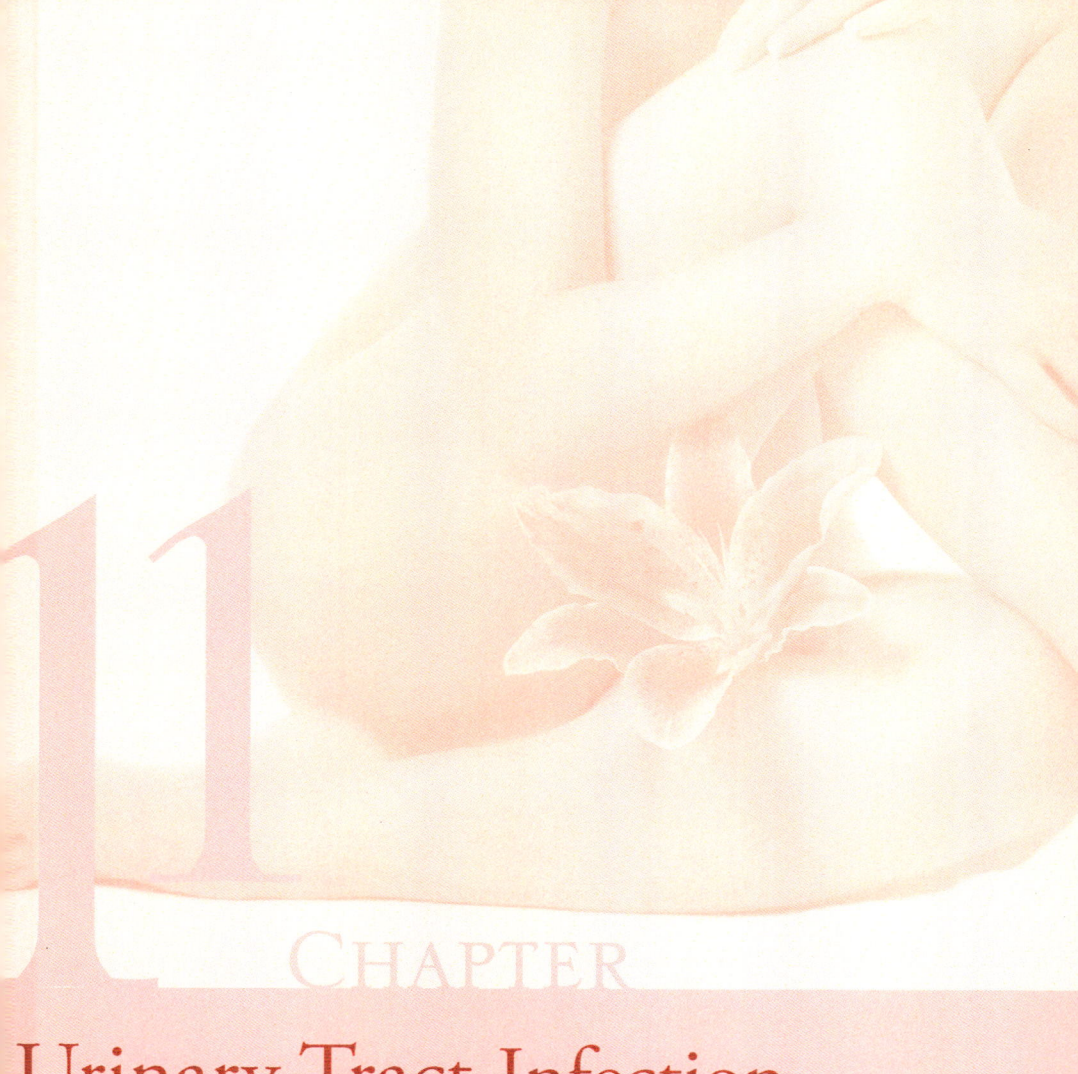

11

Urinary Tract Infection

and Recurrent
Urinary Tract Infection

"Doctor, I think I have a urine infection. Please help me."

What is Urinary Tract Infection?

A urinary tract infection (UTI) is a bacterial infection that affects any part of the urinary tract (the kidneys, ureters, bladder and urethra). Urine normally does not contain any bacteria. If bacteria get into the bladder or kidney and start to multiply, a UTI develops. Most of the time, infections are restricted to the lower urinary tract (the bladder and urethra). UTIs are very common in women, with up to 50% of them experiencing it at least once during their lifetime.

What are the Symptoms of UTI?

The common symptoms include:
• Painful urination (dysuria)
• Frequent urination (frequency)
• Frequent night-time urination (nocturia)
• Suprapubic pain
• Malodorous urine
• Haematuria
• Fever

Types of UTI

Bacteria can affect any organ in the urinary tract system, and infection of the kidney may be due to ascending infection from the bladder (Fig. 11.1).

1. Urethritis

An infection or inflammation of the urethra, causing some of the typical symptoms associated with UTI.

2. Cystitis

An infection or inflammation of the bladder, causing typical UTI symptoms.

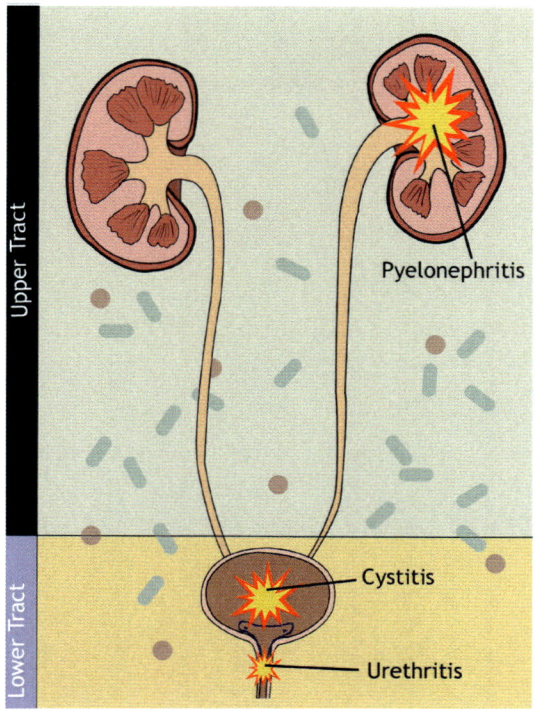

Fig. 11.1. Infection can occur throughout the entire urinary tract.

3. Acute pyelonephritis

An infection of the kidney develops when the bacterial infection spreads upwards from the bladder or through the blood stream. Symptoms include upper back pain, high fever, chills, nausea and vomiting.

What Causes UTI?

Most UTIs are caused by *Escherichia coli* (*E. coli*), a species of bacteria commonly found in the body's large bowel.

As the female urethra is close to the anus and vagina, bacteria can easily spread from the anus to the vagina and urethra. In patients with sexually transmitted diseases (STD), herpes simplex virus and bacteria such as *Chlamydia trachomatis* are possible causes of urethritis.

What are the Risk Factors for Contracting UTI?

- Women tend to get UTI much more easily than men due to the female anatomy — a shorter urethra and anal-urethral distance
- Incomplete bladder emptying increases one's risk of contracting UTI, as stale residual urine allows bacteria to rapidly multiply
- Sexual intercourse increases one's risk of contracting UTI. Certain types of spermicides can also contribute to contracting UTI
- Immunosuppressive drugs or chemotherapy leads to decrease in immunity
- Diabetes mellitus and other chronic illnesses that impair the body's immune system
- The use of tubes/catheters in the urinary tract
- Bladder or renal stones.

Screening and Diagnosis of UTI

What are the various tests used to diagnose UTI?

A urine sample (Fig. 11.2) is sent for the following tests:

- **Urinalysis** — to detect the presence of protein, sugar, blood, white blood cells and nitrites in the urine. It takes about 1 to 1½ hours before the results are ready.
- **Urine for culture and sensitivity** — this test is carried out to determine the specific bacteria or organism that is causing the infection and the most appropriate antibiotic treatment to use. Results will normally be available within a few days.

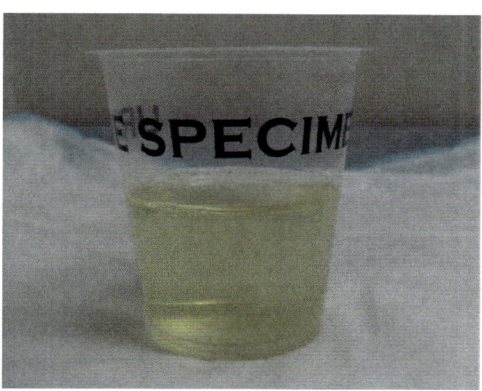

Fig. 11.2. A clean-catch urine specimen for urinalysis.

Complications

If treated promptly, a UTI usually resolves without any long-term consequences.

If left untreated or inadequately treated, the infection can spread up to the kidneys, and travel into the bloodstream, creating a slew of other problems in the body.

Treatment

Antibiotics are prescribed for simple UTI. These include amoxicilin, nitrofurantoin, bactrim or cefalexin. UTI symptoms usually subside within a few days after treatment is commenced. However, the completion of a course of antibiotics is necessary to ensure that the infection has been treated fully. Otherwise, there is a chance that resistant bacteria might grow, which may result in the patient having to be hospitalised for administration of intravenous broad spectrum antibiotics.

For recurrent infections caused by sexual activity (honeymoon cystitis), treatment involves a single dose of prescribed antibiotics, to be taken just before or after sexual intercourse.

Recurrent Urinary Tract Infection

Many women suffer from frequent UTI. When a UTI occurs three or more times in a year, it is considered as a recurrent urinary tract infection (RUTI). The RUTI may be caused by the same or different type of bacteria. Four out of five of these women may experience a new episode of infection within 18 months of the last occurence of UTI.

Symptoms

Not everyone with a UTI has symptoms, but most people have at least some symptoms to herald a new episode of infection.

These may include a frequent urge to urinate and a painful, burning feeling in the bladder or urethra during urination. It is not unusual for a person suffering from RUTI to feel tired, lethargic, and experience shaking chills and pain, so much so that she avoids urinating as much as possible. Often, women feel an uncomfortable pressure above the pubic bone. Many women with RUTI are able to tell very early on that they are getting a urine infection, and some drink more fluids to keep the infection from developing or progressing.

What are the Risk Factors for RUTI?

These are the same as those for contracting UTI (see page 96).

Investigations

Apart from urine analysis and culture, patients with RUTI may require the following additional tests:

- **Renal and pelvic ultrasound** — it is used to detect hydronephrosis (swollen kidneys), kidney and bladder stones or tumors, as well as to assess the uterus for fibroids and ovaries for cysts.
- **Cystoscopy** — a cystoscope is an instrument made of a hollow tube with several lenses and a light source, which allows the doctor to see inside the bladder through the urethra. It can be used to assess the bladder for foreign bodies, stones or tumours.
- **Urine test for cytology** — occasionally, when blood (haematuria) is persistently found on urine sample analysis, the urine specimen may be sent for checking for cancerous cells which may arise from the urinary tract.
- **Oral glucose tolerance test** — to detect diabetes mellitus.

Treatment options

The doctor may prescribe any of the following treatment options for a woman who has frequent recurrences (3 or more times a year):

- Low dose prophylactic antibiotic, such as nitrofurantoin, on a nightly basis for three months or longer. (If taken at bedtime, the drug remains in the bladder longer and may be more effective.) Studies at the University of Washington has shown this therapy to be effective without causing serious side effects.
- Single dose of appropriate antibiotic before or after sexual intercourse.
- Short course (1 or 2 days) of antibiotics when symptoms initially appear.

Preventive measures against UTI

Doctors suggest some additional steps that a woman can take on her own to avoid an infection:

Practise good personal hygiene

- Wipe from front to back to prevent bacteria around the anus from being transported to the vagina or urethra.
- Avoid using feminine hygiene sprays, scented douches, and bubble baths which may irritate the urethra. We recommend using water to wash the genital area instead.
- Cleanse the genital area before sexual intercourse.

Diet

- Drink plenty of water every day. Some doctors suggest drinking cranberry juice (Fig.11.3), which in large amounts inhibits the growth of some bacteria by acidifying the urine. Vitamin C (ascorbic acid) supplements have the same effect.
- It is best to avoid coffee, alcohol, and spicy food which may aggravate the symptoms.

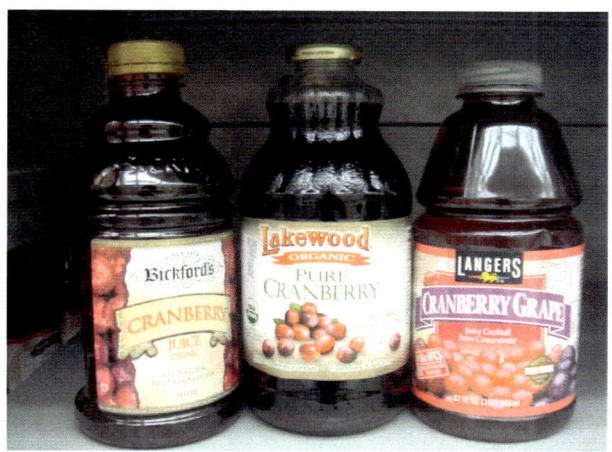

Fig. 11.3.   Cranberry juice may aid in prevention of UTI.

Other Measures

- Urinate whenever the need is felt; an urge to urinate should not be resisted.
- Pass urine before and after sexual intercourse.

Monitoring

Make an appointment with your doctor if:

- Symptoms of UTI persist even after treatment has been completed.
- Infection develops three times or more in a year.
- Symptoms worsen or new symptoms develop such as a persistent fever and back pain, while on treatment for UTI.

Conclusion

UTI can be easily treated. They may also be prevented by incorporating certain lifestyle changes. RUTI can cause great distress to the patient, if not managed aggressively and adequately. Consult your doctor or a specialist if you contract UTI.

Haematuria

"Doctor! Why am I passing blood in my urine?"

What is Haematuria?

The presence of red blood cells in the urine is known as haematuria.

What are the Different Types of Haematuria?

1. Macroscopic haematuria — Blood in the urine that is visible to the naked eye. The urine may appear red, pink or even brown.
2. Microscopic haematuria — Blood in the urine that is not visible. The presence is detected by laboratory tests like dipstick analysis (Fig. 12.1) or microscopy (Fig. 12.2).

What Causes Haematuria?

The urinary tract (Fig. 12.3) consists of the kidneys (which produce urine), the ureters (which carry urine to the bladder), the bladder (which stores urine), and the urethra (which passes urine out of the body). Diseases affecting the urinary tract system, such as bladder or kidney stones and urinary tract infections, can give rise to haematuria.

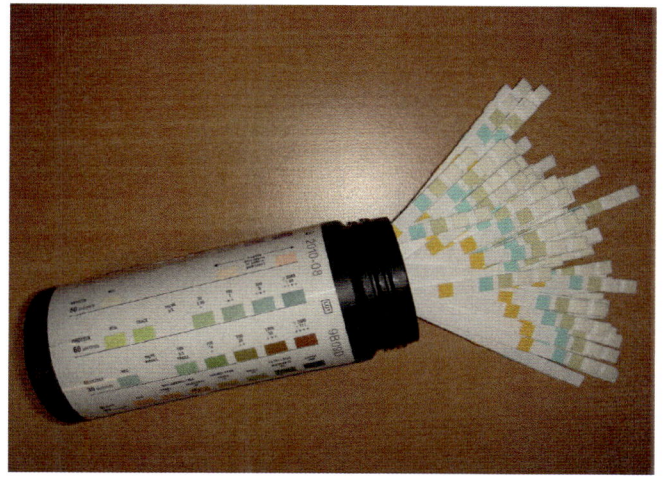

Fig. 12.1. Urine dipstick to detect the presence of red blood cells.

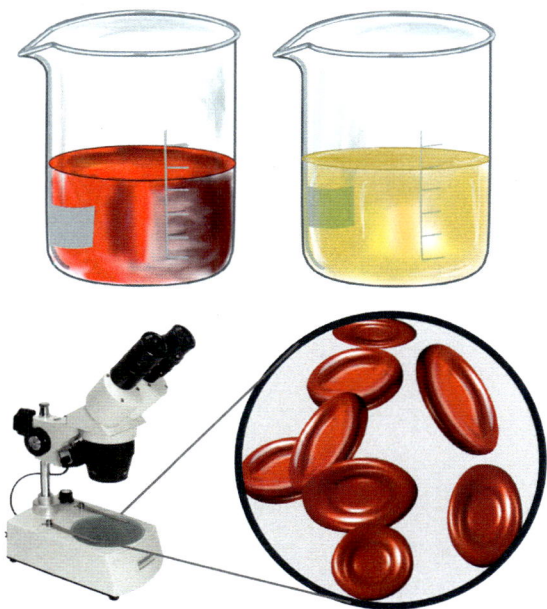

Fig. 12.2. Microscopic examination of urine for red blood cells.

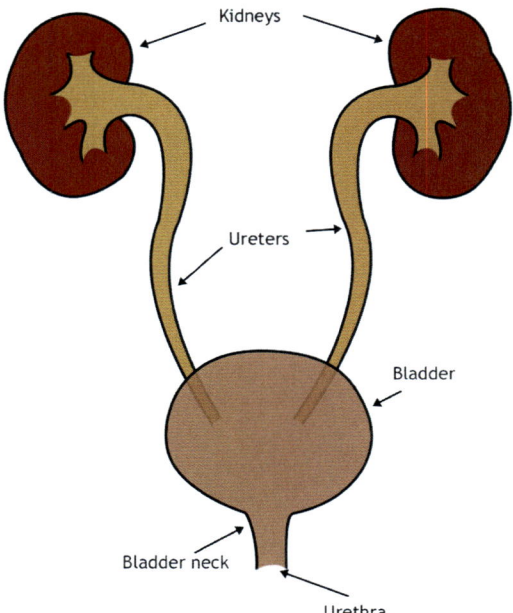

Fig. 12.3.   Diagram of the urinary tract.

Causes of haematuria

Haematuria can occur due to disease in any part of the urinary tract system. A description of causes of haematuria can be outlined as such:

1. **Kidney**

    - Stone
    - Infection (pyelonephritis)
    - Glomerulonephritis — this is a swelling of the filtering tubes (glomeruli) within the kidney. Causes include infection and immune defects of the body.
    - Tumour (growth) — this growth may be benign or cancerous. Cancer of the kidney can be painless and cause microscopic haematuria. When treated early, the prognosis is usually good.

2. **Ureter**

- Stone — can cause intense pain in the mid- and lower back that travels down to the groin (Figs. 12.4 and 12.5)
- Tumour rarely develops in the ureter

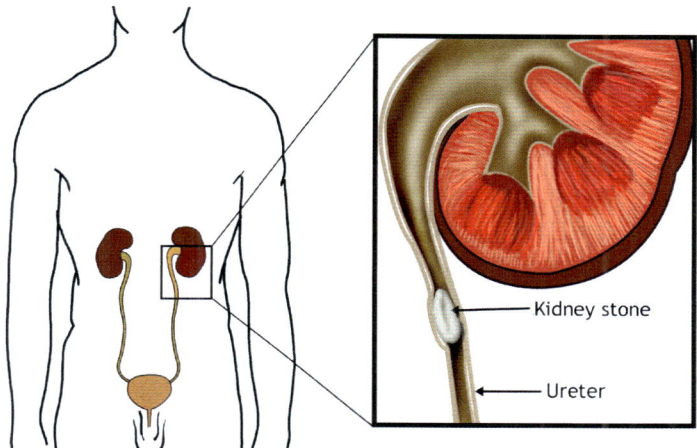

Fig. 12.4. Renal stone lodged in left ureter.

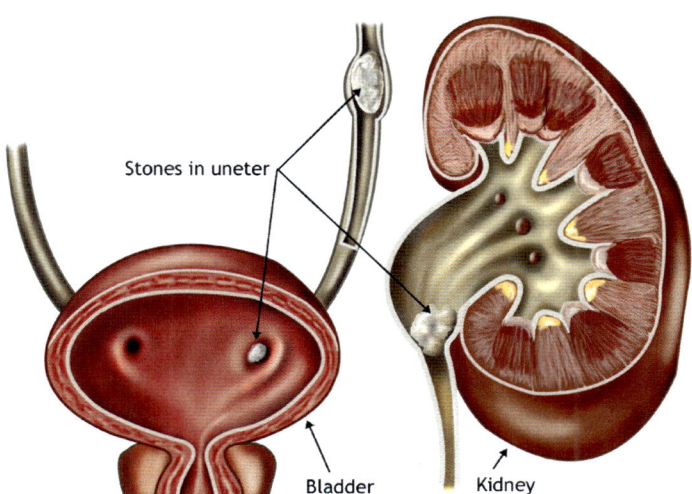

Fig. 12.5. Sites where stones are commonly located in the ureter, causing symptoms.

3. **Bladder**

- Cystitis — most commonly due to a bacterial infection. It rarely develops from exposure to radiation or noxious chemicals.
- Painful bladder syndrome (PBS) — the bladder wall is chronically inflamed. This can lead to scarring, decreased bladder capacity, bleeding, and on rare occasions, ulcers in the bladder mucosa lining.
- Stone — can occur anywhere in the urinary tract.
- Tumour — bladder cancer usually presents with gross haematuria, and may produce pain and discomfort just as in cases of cystitis.

4. **Urethra**

- Infection — this is called urethritis, and can be caused by bacteria. Infection of the urethra can also be due to sexually transmitted infections.

5. **Other causes of haematuria**

- Contamination from vaginal bleeding due to atrophic vaginitis, sexual intercourse, menstrual blood flow, or vaginal infection.
- Medical disorders, e.g. systemic lupus erythematosus (SLE), sickle cell anaemia (in which the red blood cells are more fragile and easily damaged).
- Vigorous exercise which causes local trauma as the bladder walls rub against each other.
- Physical trauma to the body can cause breakdown of muscles, leading to breakdown products that stain the urine red.
- Food, e.g. beetroot.
- Medications, e.g. aspirin.

Evaluation

When there is blood in the urine, it is necessary to seek medical help. The doctor will go through a detailed medical history so as to establish the cause of the condition.

To arrive at a diagnosis, the doctor will look out for symptoms such as urinary urgency, frequency, pain on urination, abdominal pain or fever. Doctors will also identify risk factors associated with cancer, like smoking and chemical dye exposure. After a physical examination, certain investigations and tests will be ordered.

Investigations

1. **Urine microscopy** — a raised white blood cell count in the urine may indicate the presence of a urinary tract infection (UTI), which can cause haematuria (Fig. 12.6).
2. **Urine culture** — the urine is cultured for bacteria, and if it returns positive, the sample is tested for the types of antibiotic susceptibility. This will allow the doctor to prescribe an appropriate antibiotic (Fig. 12.7).

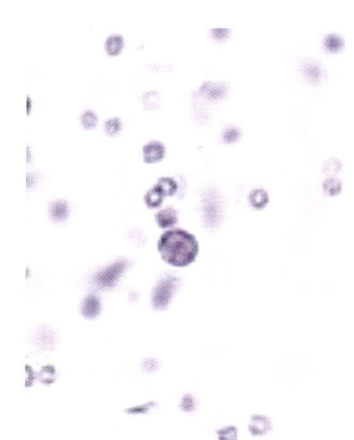

Fig. 12.6.   White blood cells in urine may indicate a UTI.

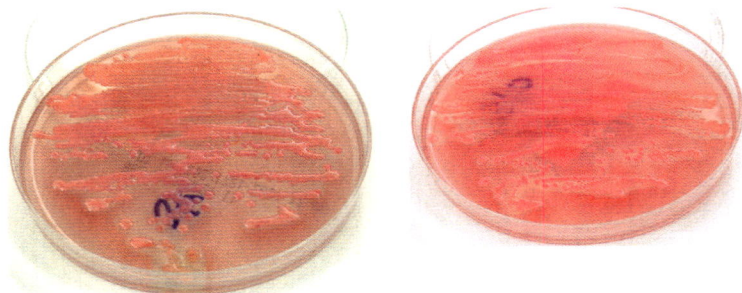

Fig. 12.7. Urine culture dishes showing bacterial growth.

3. **Urine cytology** — cells in the urine are examined to ascertain the presence of cancerous (malignant) cells, which may come from anywhere along the urinary tract. A positive finding warrants immediate attention and further evaluation (Fig. 12.8).

4. **Renal ultrasound** — this test uses ultrasound instead of radiation. The aim is to ascertain any abnormal growth in the kidney, assess the size of the kidney, and detect any abnormal swelling of the kidney and ureter (Fig. 12.9).

5. **X-ray of the kidney, ureter and bladder (KUB)** — this may help detect up to 90% of stones in the urinary tract.

6. **CT scan (CT urogram)** — computed tomography is a specialised X-ray test that examines the structure of the urinary tract. Kidney stones or masses, and abnormalities of the ureters and bladder may be detected through this method. (Fig. 12.10).

7. **Intravenous pyelogram (IVP)** — multiple X-ray films of the urinary system are taken after injection of a dye into a vein. At the end of the procedure, the patient is required to empty her bladder, before a final X-ray film is taken.

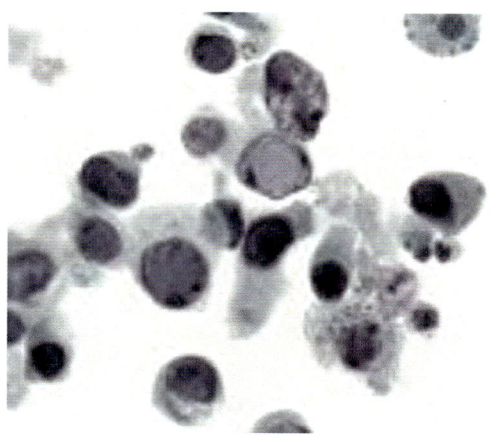

Fig. 12.8. Urine cytology revealing abnormal cancerous-looking cells of the urinary tract.

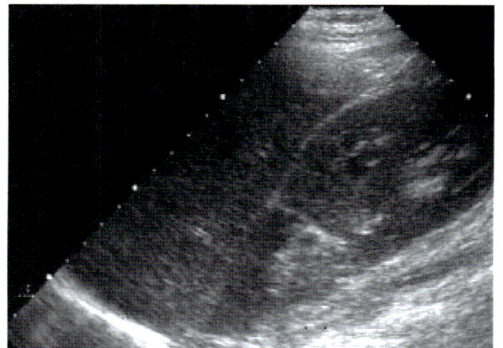 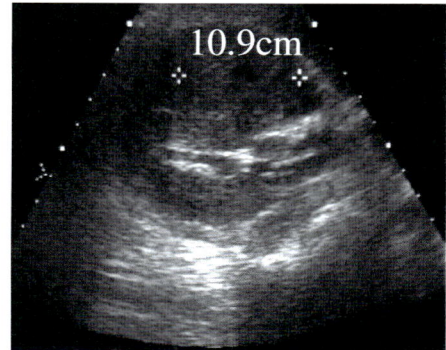

Fig. 12.9. Sonogram of normal-looking kidney.

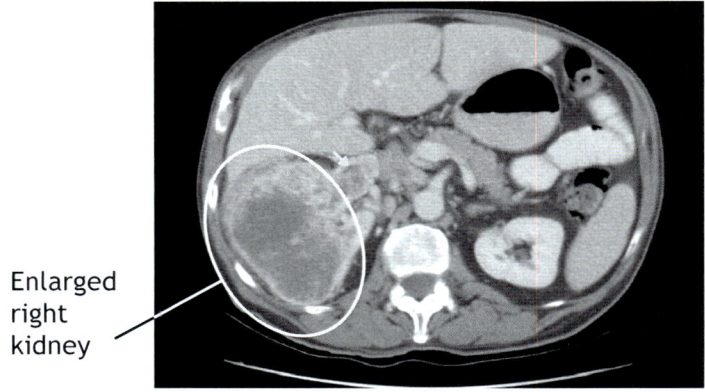

Fig. 12.10.   CT scan revealing renal cell carcinoma.

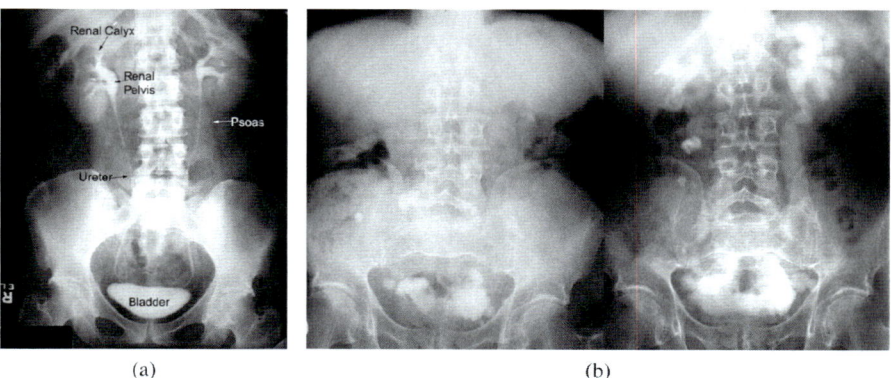

(a)   (b)

Fig. 12.11.   IVP showing (a) normal anatomy. (b) Obstruction of left ureter due to renal stone

This test detects tumours, structural abnormalities, stones or obstruction in the urinary system (Figs. 12.11a and 12.11b).

8. **Kidney biopsy** — this is a minor procedure in which a needle is used to obtain a small piece of tissue from the patient's kidney while the patient is under local anaesthesia. This sample is then checked for kidney disease such as glomerulonephritis. The information from the tissue sample is important in predicting the patient's likely progress, as well as treatment response and outcome (Fig. 12.12).

9. **Cystoscopy** — carried out while the patient is under local anaesthesia, an endoscopic camera is inserted through the urethra to examine the bladder. A biopsy may also be done during the procedure to ascertain infection, inflammation or tumour (Fig. 12.13).

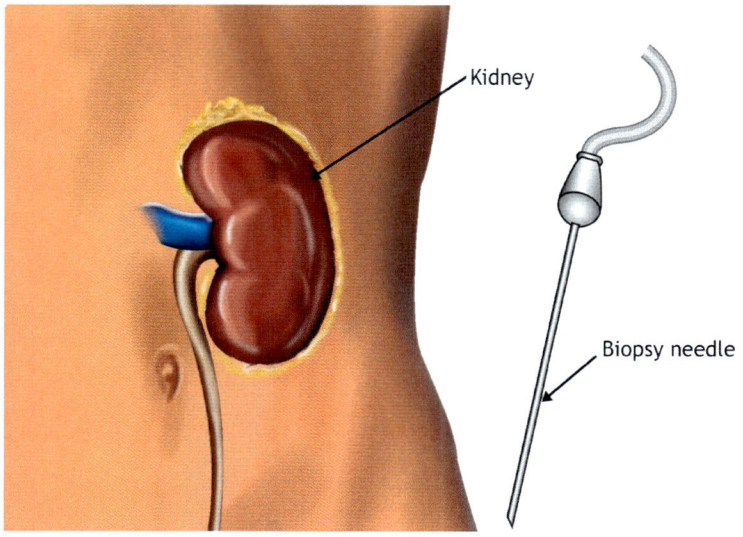

Fig. 12.12. Renal biopsy and needle used.

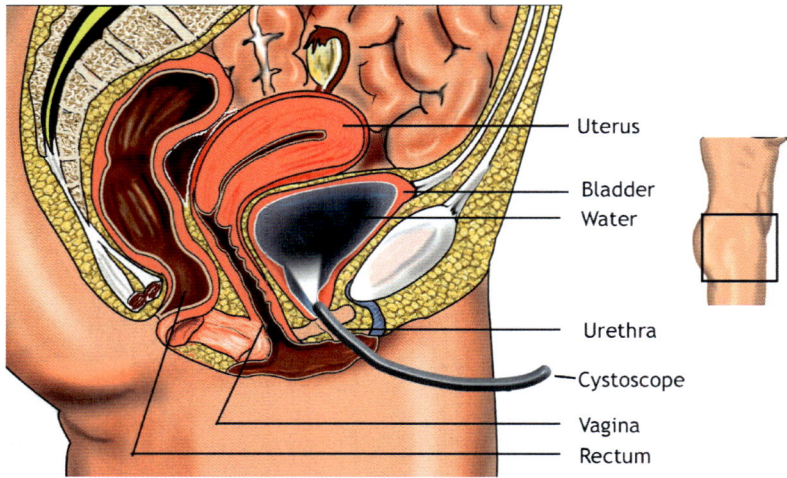

Uterus

Bladder
Water

Urethra

Cystoscope

Vagina

Rectum

Fig. 12.13.   Flexible cytoscope for examination of interior of bladder.

What is the Treatment for Haematuria?

There is no specific treatment for haematuria since it is not a disease by itself. Treatment is, however, directed at the cause of haematuria.

1. **Infection** — antibiotics and urinary antiseptics like citravescent are prescribed. It is important to practise good hygiene habits to prevent future infections (Fig. 12.14).
2. **Painful bladder syndrome** — see Chapter 10 for detailed description.
3. **Glomerulonephritis** — medications may be given to patients to manage and control the disease. In severe cases, dialysis may be required. This is managed by a renal physician (nephrologist).
4. **Stone** — treatment typically requires procedures like laser or ultrasound shockwaves to shatter urinary tract stones,

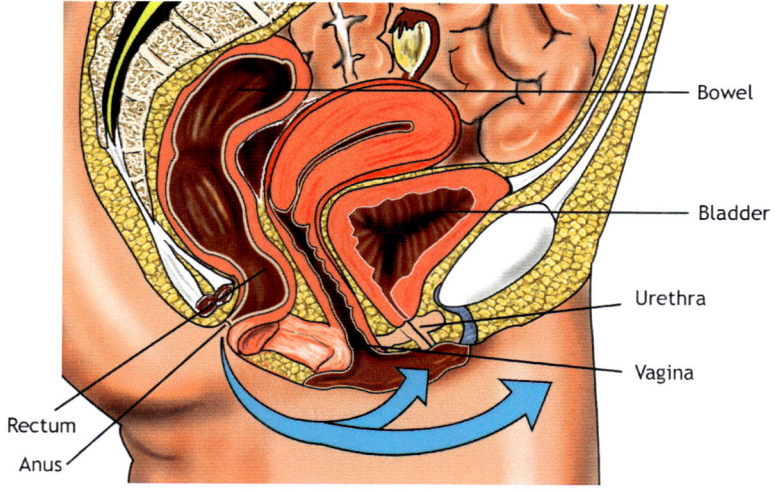

Fig. 12.14.   The wrong direction of cleaning, resulting in transfer of anal bacteria to the bladder.

as well as other measures to prevent a recurrence. This is usually managed by a urologist.

5. **Cancer** — this requires surgical removal of the tumour. In addition, chemotherapy or radiotherapy may be required. A referral to our urology colleagues is required.

6. **Medications** — medications should be discontinued if possible.

7. **Trauma** — treatment is prescribed according to severity of injury, ranging from bed rest and close observation to surgical repair and the removal of the damaged tissue or organ in severe cases.

Conclusion

Haematuria is an alarming condition for most patients whenever it occurs. The first course of action is not to panic but to seek professional help to ascertain the cause of the haematuria, and have it treated as soon as possible so as to ensure a good outcome.

Ageing and Urogenital Syndrome

"Doctor, I don't feel very comfortable below..."

What is Urogenital Syndrome and What are Its Symptoms?

Urogenital syndrome is a term that describes vaginal and urinary symptoms caused by oestrogen deficiency. It is a condition that is associated with menopause, or after the surgical removal of ovaries (oophorectomy).

The vaginal symptoms include:

- Dryness
- Soreness
- Itching
- Painful sexual intercourse (dyspareunia)
- Superficial vaginal bleeding
- Vaginal discharge secondary to infection

The urinary symptoms include:

- Pain when passing urine (dysuria)
- Frequent urination (frequency)
- Sudden and overwhelming need to pass urine (urgency)
- Urinary leakage associated with sensation of urgency (urge incontinence)
- Recurrent urinary tract infections (RUTI)

Urogenital complaints are very common in menopausal women and these symptoms can cause considerable suffering, and lead to a reduced quality of life.

What Happens to the Urogenital Tract after Menopause?

The urogenital tract is made up of the pelvic floor muscles, bladder, urine tube (urethra), and the vagina. Oestrogen receptors are found in the vagina, urethra, bladder, and pelvic muscles.

After menopause:

- The lack of oestrogen causes degenerative changes to the urogenital tissues.
- The vaginal opening becomes narrower and the vagina shortens.
- The outer vaginal walls appear pale, smooth, shiny and dry (atrophic).
- The vaginal pH level increases (more alkaline) such that organisms predisposing to vaginal infections replace healthy vaginal flora.
- Atrophic changes in the urethra and bladder predispose a woman to urinary symptoms.
- The pelvic floor tissues and ligaments lose their strength and elasticity, causing prolapse symptoms.
- Other factors may also contribute to urinary incontinence. They include hereditary factors, obesity and previous childbirth.

What are the Treatment Options?

It is important to seek advice from a doctor as vaginal infection, UTI, tissue irritation from incontinence or the use of harsh feminine hygiene products, can result in similar symptoms or aggravate existing urogenital syndrome.

Urogenital symptoms vary widely. Hence, when prescribing treatment, doctors need to take into account the troublesome symptoms, the patient's lifestyle and risk factors.

The therapeutic options include both non-hormonal and hormonal treatments, or combination therapy.

What Simple Measures can be Taken to Relieve Troublesome Symptoms?

Certain lifestyle changes can help reduce the severity of symptoms.

They include:

- Adequate fluid intake
- Wearing loose clothing
- Avoiding vaginal douching or use of vaginal feminine products
- Using vaginal lubricants and moisturisers such as Replens

At the same time, patients should bear in mind that:

- There is no strong evidence that phytoestrogens or herbal supplements provide any benefit to relieve the symptoms of urogenital syndrome.
- There is some evidence that drinking cranberry or lingonberry juice can reduce one's chance of contracting UTI.

How Can Oestrogen Hormonal Treatment Help?

The urogenital tract responds to oestrogen therapy which is used in the treatment of vaginal atrophy. This form of treatment also benefits those who suffer from frequency, urgency, and urgency urinary incontinence.

Oestrogen therapy has been shown to:

- Increase cellular regeneration in the vagina, bladder and urethra
- Re-acidify the vagina and reverse menopause-associated microbiological changes.
- Improve continence by increasing urethral resistance and increasing bladder volume such that the bladder can contain more urine before the desire to urinate is triggered.

What are the types of oestrogen therapy available?

Oestrogen therapy can be administered as tablets (orally), in the form of a skin patch or gel (transdermally), or vaginally (conjugated equine oestrogen cream, oestradiol cream, oestradiol tablets or pessaries, and oestradiol-releasing ring). The various modes differ in terms of delivery, dosage, and the amount of oestrogen absorbed through the bloodstream.

When should oestrogen therapy be avoided?

Patients should not be prescribed oestrogen if they have the following:

- Abnormal vaginal bleeding
- Breast cancer
- History of endometrial cancer
- History of blood clots (*thromboembolic disease*)
- Pregnancy
- Breastfeeding

Oestrogen therapy should be used with caution in patients who have impaired liver function or heart disease.

Women who experience post-menopausal bleeding after being started on oestrogen therapy must stop the treatment and seek medical attention immediately.

Which Hormone Replacement Therapy (HRT) is Best for the Treatment of Urogenital Syndrome?

Oral or transdermal hormone replacement therapy

Oral or transdermal hormone replacement therapy (HRT) is useful in patients experiencing menopausal symptoms. However, many women will still experience urogenital symptoms despite being on HRT.

The possible systemic side effects include:
• Headache
• Breast tenderness or pain
• Perineal discomfort or pain
• Vaginal bleeding
• Possible increased risk of an oestrogen-dependent tumour

As such, the systemic routes of delivery do not benefit patients whose main complaint is that of urogenital syndrome. In addition, significant side effects make systemic HRT a less suitable treatment modality.

Vaginal oestrogen preparations

The vaginal route of oestrogen delivery is the preferred treatment route, as it is not only effective, it also avoids systemic side effects.

In using topical therapy, only a lower dose of oestrogen is required for symptom relief as compared with systemic HRT. Treatment is usually short-term (up to 3 months) and is safe for women who still have their uterus.

Vaginal oestrogen cream

This comes in the form of oestradiol cream. The cream is inserted vaginally once a day, and after 2 weeks, reduced to twice a week to achieve symptom control. Oestrogen creams should be used at the lowest effective dose as it can still be absorbed through the vaginal skin, resulting in undesired systemic side effects.

Vaginal oestradiol pessary

With the aid of an applicator, one pessary is inserted into the vagina daily for two weeks, after which the dose is reduced to one tablet twice a week. This dosage schedule limits the systemic absorption of oestradiol while allowing for the effective treatment of atrophic symptoms.

Vaginal oestradiol-releasing ring (Estring)

A flexible silicone ring containing 17 beta-oestradiol, is inserted into the vagina, and remains in place for three months. The ring provides a continuous release of oestradiol which is minimally absorbed systematically.

There is no need to remove the ring during activities such as bathing or sexual intercourse, although some women may choose to do so. In these circumstances, the ring may be rinsed with water before being reinserted into the vagina. Women who find it difficult to reinsert the device into the vagina can approach their doctor for help. A new pessary can be inserted depending on the doctor's discretion and judgement.

Conclusion

Although urogenital syndrome is a natural consequence of declining oestrogen levels, its symptoms nevertheless significantly impair a patient's quality of life. Various topical oestrogen products, in addition to over-the-counter vaginal moisturisers, provide effective treatment options to reduce symptoms, and uphold patients' quality of life through their golden years.

14

Urinary Incontinence Aids

Pads, Catheters and Care for Urinary Aids

Incontinence aids are products specifically developed to allow women to maintain continence, lessen discomfort, increase confidence and keep their dignity.

These products benefit those women who, in spite of having undergone other treatments, still remain incontinent; are too ill, unsuitable for surgery, refuse surgery, or are awaiting continence surgery.

Absorbent Continence Pads

Unlike sanitary napkin, continence pads are designed to absorb and hold urine without leakage until the next change. A pad should fit well and be able to prevent odour.

A basic pad is made up of three layers:

1. Waterproof backing — to prevent clothing from becoming wet or stained.
2. Middle absorbent layer — usually made of layers of cellulose fibres. Super-absorbent powders may be added to the middle layer to make it thinner, less bulky, and capable of absorbing large amounts of urine.
3. Cover stock — the layer touching the skin is usually designed to prevent urine from coming in contact with the skin. It is made of biodegradable, hydrophobic fibres which prevents skin problems or reactions due to prolonged contact with urine.

Pads come in many sizes, styles and absorbency levels (Fig. 14.1). The choice of the type of pad depends on the degree of incontinence a patient suffers from.

A small plastic-backed pad placed in a normal underwear is able to hold urine of not more than 50 ml. However, for larger volumes of urine loss, a thicker and more absorbent pad is needed. These pads are kept in place by self-adhesive tapes.

All-in-one diapers are suitable for those with severe urinary or faecal incontinence and also for patients who are less mobile or are bedridden.

An increasingly popular product is the disposable pull-up pants (Fig. 14.2). It is convenient, not conspicuous and does not restrict one's choice of clothing. It also allows the wearer to use the toilet normally.

The absorbent bed pad is a product suitable for use on its own or as an additional protective layer for bedlinen and the mattress. It is designed as a rectangular sheet, has a waterproof non-slip backing, an absorbent centre with fluid-dispersing properties and a non-woven stay-dry top layer.

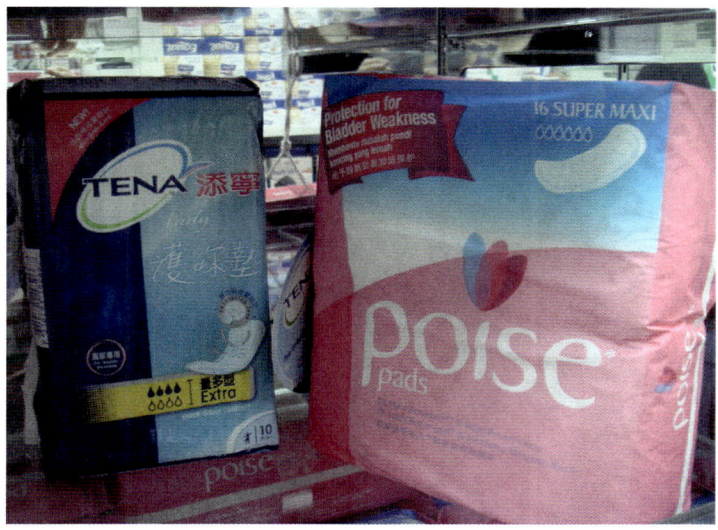

Fig. 14.1.   Different brands of continence pads.

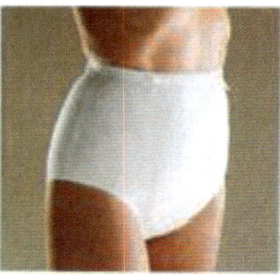

POWERFUL PROTECTION

The **New** Alternative to Bulky Guards and Undergarments

light to moderate protection

Fig. 14.2.   "Panty-styled" continence pad.

When absorbent products are used, the practice of good hygiene and frequent pad changes are required to prevent skin irritation and the risk of UTI.

Urinary Catheters

A urinary catheter is a tube that is inserted into the bladder through the urethra in order to drain urine.

Catheters come in many sizes and are made of different materials (Fig. 14.3). Some catheters are designed for short-term and others for long-term use.

Catheters for short-term use

These catheters can be made of plastic or PVC, latex or Teflon-coated latex.

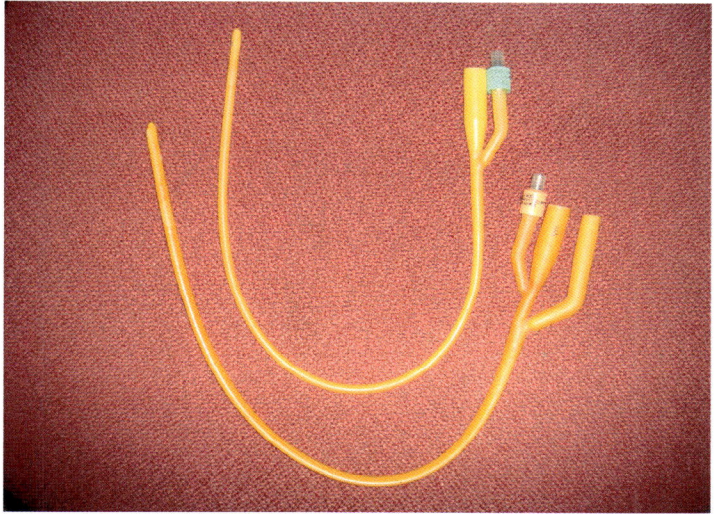

Fig. 14.3. Different types of urinary catheters.

A plastic or PVC catheter has thin walls and a wide internal diameter. It is a stiff catheter and is usually used for intermittent (non-continuous or one-use only) catheterisation.

Latex is the most commonly used material. A latex catheter is flexible and can be used as a self-retaining catheter (i.e. for securing inside the body) for up to 14 days.

A Teflon-coated latex catheter is also a self-retaining catheter and can remain in place for up to 28 days.

Catheters for long-term use

A pure silicone catheter is less likely to cause bodily discomfort and can remain in place for longer periods of up to 12 weeks.

Catheter size ranges from 8 FG to 30 FG (French Gauge) and catheter length varies in length from 16 cm to 25 cm for female, and 40 cm to 46 cm for male.

All self-retaining catheters are secured in place by a tiny balloon.

After the catheter is inserted into the bladder, a carefully measured volume (about 5 ml to 7 ml) of sterile water is syringed into the balloon-inflation channel of the catheter. This causes the balloon to expand and keeps the catheter in place, preventing it from slipping out of the bladder (Fig. 14.4a & b).

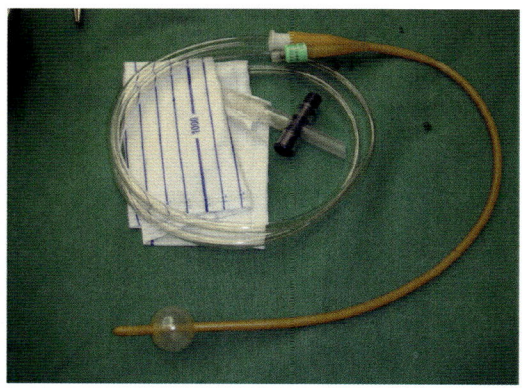

Fig. 14.4a. Catheter and urine bag set-up.

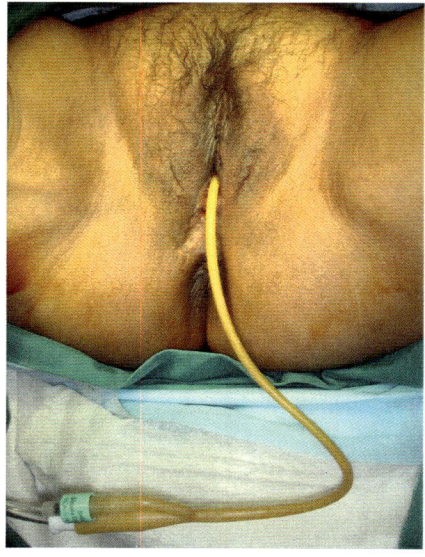

Fig. 14.4b. Catheter in-situ after operation.

When the time comes for the catheter to be removed, the water is drawn out from the balloon. Then the catheter can be easily removed from the bladder.

It is recommended that a suitably sized catheter be used depending on the clinical situation. Some patients may require a larger catheter if their urine contain blood clot or sediment, which may block smaller catheters. Studies have shown that a catheter size of 12 to 14 is usually sufficient to drain the urine produced by an adult.

15

CHAPTER

Pelvic Floor Exercises

Pelvic floor exercises (PFE) are a regime of pelvic muscle exercises designed to improve the muscle tone of the pelvic floor.

The principle behind PFE is to strengthen the muscles of the pelvic floor, with the aim of improving the body's urethral and rectal sphincter functions. The success of PFE depends on the use of proper technique and adherence to a regular, long-term exercise programme.

Some people have difficulty identifying their pelvic floor muscles. Care must be taken when flexing these muscles, as an incorrect technique may worsen pelvic floor tone, pelvic organ prolapse and urinary incontinence — some people contract the abdominal or thigh muscles, and not the pelvic floor muscles.

There are several methods to help one identify the pelvic floor muscles. One way to do this is when one is clearing the bowels — half-way through defaecating — the patient could stop the passage of motion by contracting the pelvic floor muscles. She could repeat this several times until she is aware of the flexing of the correct muscle group. Another way is to stop her urine flow mid-stream when urinating. In this way, the patient becomes aware of the pelvic floor muscles and how to contract them.

Another approach is by inserting a finger into the vagina, and tightening the muscles around the finger, as if holding back urine. During this exercise, the abdominal and thigh muscles should remain relaxed.

A woman may also strengthen her pelvic floor muscles with the use of a set of graduated weights (vaginal cones) which she tries to hold in her vagina (Fig. 15.1).

Other methods such as biofeedback and electrical stimulation may also help one identify the pelvic floor muscles.

Biofeedback is a method of positive reinforcement. Electrodes are placed on the abdomen and the anal area. Some therapists place a sensor in either a woman's vagina or a man's anus, so as to monitor pelvic floor muscle contractions. A computer-generated graph will then indicate which muscles are correctly contracting and which are at rest.

Electrical stimulation involves using a low-voltage electric current to stimulate the correct group of muscles. The current is delivered using an anal or vaginal probe and the electrical stimulation therapy may be performed in a clinic or at home. Treatment sessions usually take 20 minutes and may be held over a one to four-day period of time. So far, this method has shown promising results when treating patients with stress and urge incontinence.

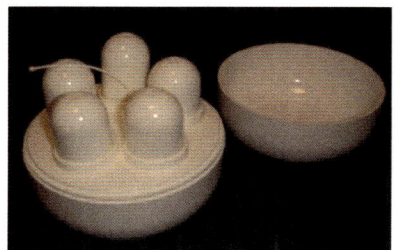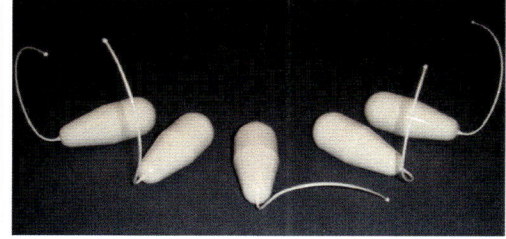

Fig. 15.1. A set of vaginal cones.

Performing Pelvic Floor Exercises

- Tighten the pelvic floor muscles and hold to the count of 10.
- Relax the muscles to the count of 10.
- Perform 10 sets of squeezes, three times a day (morning, afternoon and night).

These exercises can be performed at any time and at any place. Most people attempt them lying down or sitting on a chair. In just four to six weeks, most people begin to notice some improvements in their condition, although it may take up to three months for a significant change. It has been shown that PFE, if carried out properly, could improve urinary incontinence symptoms by up to 60%.

Some people believe they can improve their condition significantly by increasing the frequency of pelvic floor exercises. However, over-exercising can lead to muscle fatigue and worsen urinary leakage.

Performing PFE incorrectly can also result in discomfort in the abdomen or back area. Some people have a tendency to hold their breath or tense up when contracting the pelvic floor muscles. It is important to relax and focus on exercising only the pelvic floor muscles.

16

Where to Seek Professional Help and Advice?

There are many doctors who could help patients who have urinary and pelvic organ prolapse problems. These include family physicians, medical specialists and gynaecologists. There are specialists who sub-specialise in this field, namely urologists with an interest in female urology and urogynaecologists. Do not be afraid to contact any of these doctors if you need to seek help.

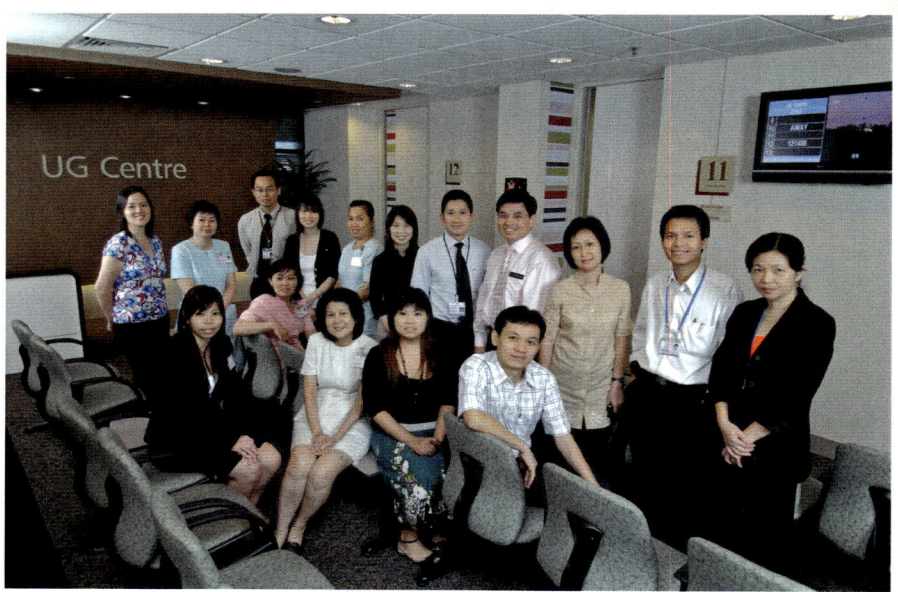

Our team of professional medical staff includes specialists, and nurse practitioners. Department of Urogynaecology, KK Women's & Children's Hospital.

Our Full-time Doctors include:

Adj. Associate Professor William Han How Chuan

MBBS (Singapore), FRCOG (London),
MMED (O&G) (Singapore),
HMDP in Urogynaecology (London), FAMS (O&G)
Obstetrician & Gynaecologist
Head & Senior Consultant, Urogynaecology Surgery Unit,
Head, Department of Urogynaecology
KK Women's & Children's Hospital

Adj. Assistant Professor Dr Lee Lih Charn

MBBS (Singapore), MMED (O&G), FAMS (O&G)
HMDP in Urogynaecology (Australia)
Obstetrician & Gynaecologist
Head & Senior Consultant, Ambulatory Care &
Urodynamics Unit, Department of Urogynaecology
KK Women's & Children's Hospital

Dr Arthur Tseng Leng Aun

MBChB Honours (Sheffield), MRCOG (London),
HMDP in Urogynaecology (London)
Obstetrician & Gynaecologist
Consultant, Department of Urogynaecology
KK Women's & Children's Hospital

Dr Wong Heng Fok

MBBS (Singapore), MRCOG (London)
Obstetrician & Gynaecologist
Associate Consultant, Department of Urogynaecology
KK Women's & Children's Hospital

Our Visiting Specialist include:

Dr Christopher Chong

MBBS, MMED (O&G), MRCOG (London),
Visiting Specialist, Department of Urogynaecology

For enquiries, please contact:

KK Urogynaecology Centre
Tel: 65 6394 1491/ 1492/ 1493/ 1494
Fax: 65 6394 1448

To make an appointment:

KKH Appointment Services
Tel: 65 6294 4050

Glossary

Abdomen The part of the body between the thorax (chest) and pelvis

Antibiotics A substance produced by or derived from certain fungi, bacteria and other organisms, that can destroy or inhibit the growth of other micro-organisms. Examples are penicillin and streptomycin

Aspiration The act of inhaling fluid or a foreign body into the bronchi and lungs, often after vomiting

Atrophy The state of wasting away or deterioration

Autoimmune Destruction of an organ or system by the body's own defences

Biofeedback A method of learning to control one's bodily functions by recognising and changing it through visual signals that represent a normally unconscious process. Bladder diaries are a form of biofeedback

Bladder	A sac-shaped muscular organ in the pelvis that stores the urine produced by the kidneys
Cardiac	Relating to or involving the heart
Catheter	A hollow flexible tube inserted into a body cavity, duct or vessel to facilitate the movement of bodily fluids or distend a passageway
Chondriotin sulphate	An important structural component of cartilage which provides much of its shock absorbent properties. Also found in the bladder GAG layer.
Chronic	Relating to an illness or medical condition that is characterised by a long duration or frequent recurrence
Compliance	The act of conforming, acquiescing, yielding, or physically relaxing
Conservative	Utilizing other treatment modalities like lifestyle changes, physical therapies or medications, instead of surgical means of treatment.
Constipation	A condition of the bowels in which the faeces are dry and hard, leading to difficult and infrequent bowel movements
Continence	The ability to control urinary and faecal discharge
Contrast	A type of dye
Cyst	An abnormal membranous sac containing liquid or semisolid substance

Cystocoele	Prolapse of the bladder through the front wall of the vagina
Diuretic	A substance or drug to increase the production of urine; it is frequently used to control hypertension or heart failure
Dribbling	A small trickling stream associated with voiding difficulty
Dysuria	Pain when passing urine
Empirical	Derived from trial and error experimentation, rather than from theory and standardised testing
Erosion	The state of being worn away or broken down
Frequency	Frequent urination (>7 times/day)
Fibroid	A benign tumour composed of fibrous or muscle tissue that develops in the uterus
GAG layer	Protective coating in the bladder
Haematuria	Blood in urine
Herniating	To protrude abnormally from an enclosed cavity or from the body
Hydronephrosis	Swelling of the kidney
Hydroureter	Swelling of the ureter
Hypoxia	Lack of oxygen
Hysterectomy	Surgical removal of the womb (uterus)
Inflammation	A response of bodily tissue to injury or irritation which is characterised by pain, swelling and redness

Ligament	A sheet or band of tough, fibrous tissue connecting bones or cartilages at a joint or supporting an organ
Lumbar	The part of the back between the ribs and the hips
Mast cell	One of the cell types that make up part of our immunologic defence
Menopausal	The period marked by the natural and permanent cessation of menstruation, occurring usually between the ages of 45 and 55 years
Nocturia	Abnormal urination at night (≥ 1 time per night)
Obstetric	Pertaining to the care and treatment of women before, during and after childbirth
Oestrogen	Female reproductive hormone
Ovaries	The female gonad or reproductive organ
Perineum	The region between the anus and the genital opening (vagina)
Pessary	A device worn in the vagina to support a displaced uterus
Prolapse	The downward displacement of an organ or part of it from its normal position
Radiation	The treatment of disease (especially cancer) by exposure to a radioactive source
Rectocoele	Herniation of part of the rectum through the back wall of the vagina

Rectum	The end portion of the large intestine, extending from the sigmoid colon to the anal canal
Recurrent	Occurring again or repeatedly
Residual	Remaining in an organ or part following normal discharge or expulsion
Retention	The state or action of keeping a fluid or secretion in a body cavity
Sacrum	A triangular bone made up of five fused bones and forming the posterior section of the pelvis
Saline	An isotonic solution of sodium chloride and distilled water
Stricture	An abnormal contraction of any passage or duct of the body
Suprapubic	Above the pubic bone
TED	Thrombo-embolic deterrent (stockings), a method of preventing blood clots from developing in the calf muscle veins
Ulcer	A break in the skin
Urethra	The muscular tube that extends from the urinary bladder to the exterior of the body
Urgency	Sudden and overwhelming need to pass urine that is difficult to defer
Urotoxins	Noxious substances that cause irritation or damage to the urinary tract system
UTI	Urinary tract infection
Voiding	The act of emptying the bladder

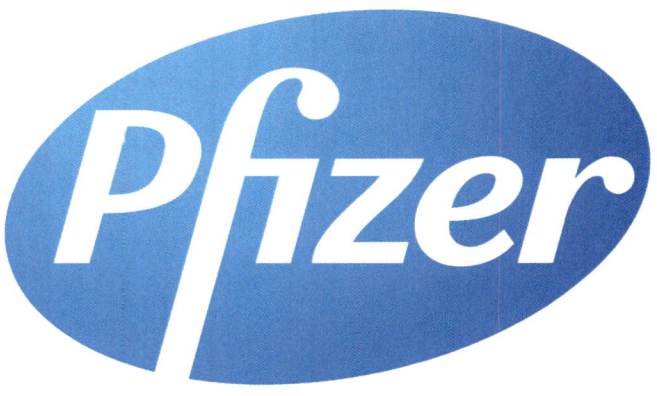
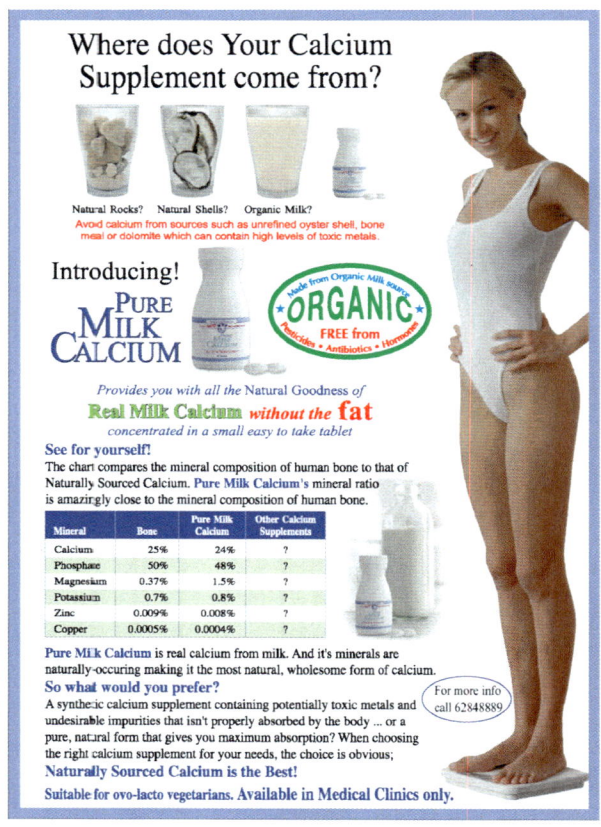

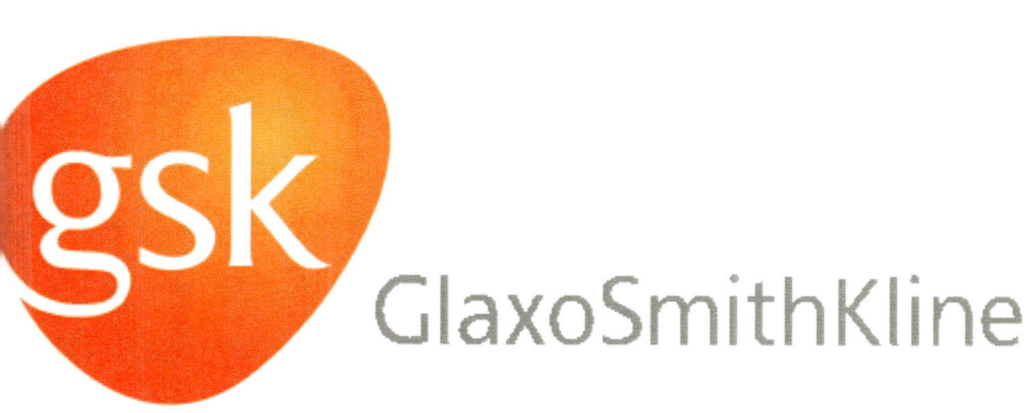

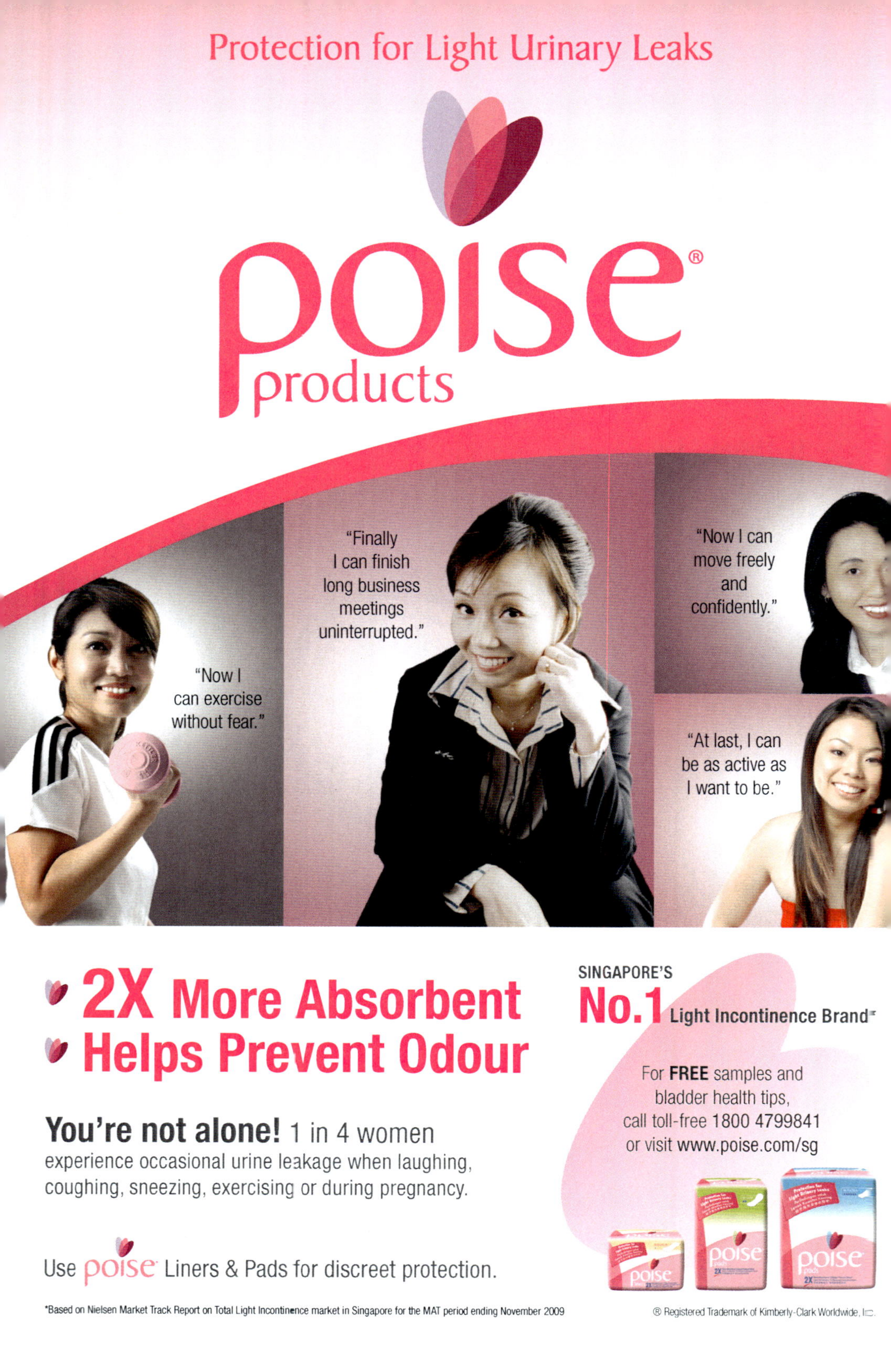

Protection for Light Urinary Leaks

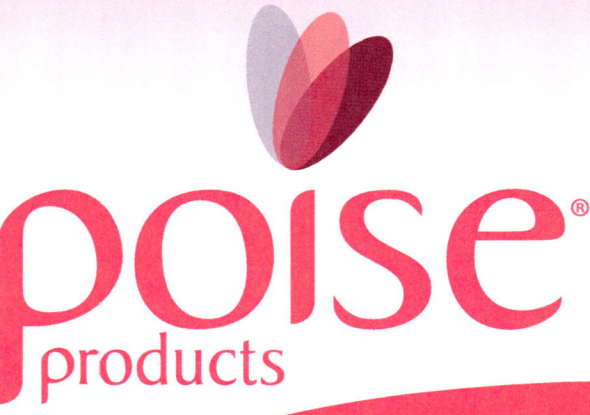

poise® products

"Finally I can finish long business meetings uninterrupted."

"Now I can exercise without fear."

"Now I can move freely and confidently."

"At last, I can be as active as I want to be."

❤ 2X More Absorbent
❤ Helps Prevent Odour

You're not alone! 1 in 4 women experience occasional urine leakage when laughing, coughing, sneezing, exercising or during pregnancy.

Use poise Liners & Pads for discreet protection.

SINGAPORE'S
No.1 Light Incontinence Brand*

For **FREE** samples and bladder health tips, call toll-free 1800 4799841 or visit www.poise.com/sg

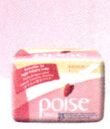
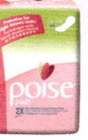
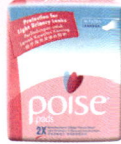

*Based on Nielsen Market Track Report on Total Light Incontinence market in Singapore for the MAT period ending November 2009

® Registered Trademark of Kimberly-Clark Worldwide, Inc.

Made in United States
Orlando, FL
22 March 2026

79557572R00100